SPORTS MASSAGE
AND STRETCHING

Acknowledgements

For the photography in this book thanks go to David McClenaghan.
Copyright on all photos retained by the Australian Institute of Sport.

SPORTS MASSAGE
AND STRETCHING

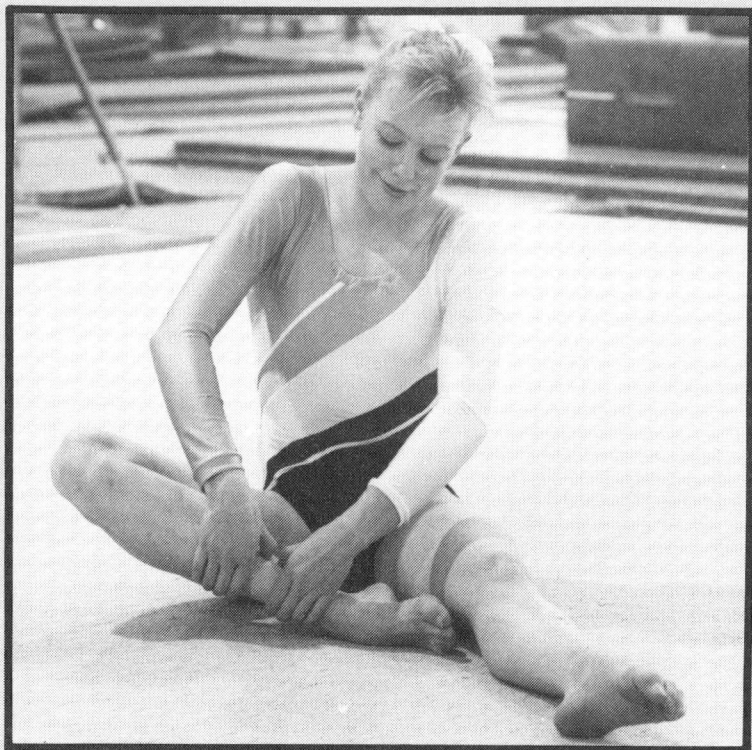

WAYDE CLEWS

PARTRIDGE PRESS

LONDON · NEW YORK · TORONTO · SYDNEY · AUCKLAND

Dedication

To my wife Cherylynne and my parents Marlene and Tom.

SPORTS MASSAGE AND STRETCHING

PARTRIDGE PRESS

Published by Partridge Press 1990
a division of TRANSWORLD PUBLISHERS LTD
61-63 Uxbridge Road, London W5 5SA,
TRANSWORLD PUBLISHERS (AUSTRALIA) PTY LTD
15-25 Helles Avenue, Moorebank, NSW 2170,
TRANSWORLD PUBLISHERS (NZ) LTD
Cnr Moselle and Waipareira Avenues,
Henderson, Auckland.

Copyright © Wayde Clews

British Library Cataloguing in Publication Data
Clews, Wayde

  Sports massage and stretching.
  1. Physical fitness. Massage
  I. Title
  613.79

ISBN 1-85225-120-4

Typeset in Australia by Excel Imaging
Printed in Australia by The Book Printer

Cover designed by Wing Ping Tong
Text designed by Trevor Hood

CONTENTS

FOREWORD

I never fully appreciated the importance of massage in aiding athletic performance and recovery until Wayde Clews introduced me to massage therapy in the early 1980s. Since then, however, it has become a vital part of my training and competitive preparation.

I first met Wayde in 1974 at the Australian Cross Country Championships, held in Perth, Western Australia. Wayde was eleven years old when he and his sister approached me for my autograph after I finished second in the under-19 championship. I eagerly obliged, not having signed many autographs before. I remember writing 'with grateful thanks' and then signing my name. I am grateful for that meeting, because some six years later I married his sister and three years after that Wayde became my regular masseur.

After qualifying as a teacher and working for a while for the Western Australian Education Department, Wayde began to study massage therapy in order to help many of his athlete friends who were plagued by injuries. (His own promising athletic career had ended abruptly with a serious knee injury.) At first he helped as many people as he could while continuing to teach, but eventually the demand for his services warranted his leaving teaching to devote himself to sports massage.

Since then Wayde has contributed greatly to my athletic success . He massages me twice a week when I am training in Australia, and has accompanied me to several major international competitions, where I have found his services indispensable.

Wayde has worked with world-ranked Australian and international athletes, as well as treating many prominent public figures, including our Prime Minister, Mr Bob Hawke.

Most of the athletes from a wide variety of sports who have passed through the Australian Institute of Sport (AIS) in Canberra, where Wayde has worked since 1984, acknowledge the benefit they have received from his treatment methods. Consequently his talents have been in great demand. In the process, he has devised a comprehensive solution to many problems associated with sporting injury and maintenance of physical fitness.

Wayde's solution lies in his development of 'self-massage techniques' which individuals engaging in sport at a recreational, community or even top competitive level can employ themselves, either because they may not have access to regular massage for financial or other reasons, or simply because the masseur available is not specifically trained in the skills of sports massage.

Being a qualified and competent educator has enabled Wayde to contribute the knowledge of not only his own skills but the needs of athletes and the knowledge of other members of the sports medicine staff at the AIS in designing this program, which can help both with recovery from strenuous exercise and the prevention of athletic injuries.

If employed correctly and on a regular basis, 'self-massage' could become as recognised in aiding recovery from exercise and the prevention of trauma as stretching before and after physical activity is now.

This simply-illustrated book is a wonderful manual for athletes, coaches, sports medicine practitioners and physical educators interested in the wellbeing of their pupils.

I recommend it highly.

Robert de Castella

INTRODUCTION

Every sportsperson has individual goals and ambitions which may range from completing a fun-run distance to winning gold at the Olympic Games. The one common aim for everybody involved in sport is the desire to perform at the very best of their ability and in doing so realise their full potential.

Assuming that your training, mental approach and lifestyle are all aimed at optimal performance, the greatest barrier to reaching your real potential, however, will more than likely be injury.

This book presents an approach by which both the dedicated athlete and the recreational sportsperson can enhance performance by preventing injury and facilitating quicker recovery.

Intensive training workloads put the body under great stress and without appropriate care and management, enforced periods of reduction in the effort and frequency of training may be a stumbling block in your preparation.

Many of us neglect or ignore the needs of our bodies and, sadly, some tried and true methods for enhancing performance, preventing injury and promoting quicker recovery are not understood.

It is widely accepted that massage is a valuable adjunct to any sportsperson's training regime. Massage fulfils many roles throughout an athlete's preparation, including facilitating quicker recovery and adaptation during heavy workloads. It is used in the prevention and treatment of a diverse range of soft tissue and associated injuries. Just as importantly, relaxation massage helps athletes cope with the many stresses resulting from the highly disciplined lives they lead. Massage also plays a vital part in the last phase of preparation, immediately prior to competition.

Athletes who have had some experience of massage and realised its benefits invariably try to make it an integral part of their training programs.

Working as a masseur at the Australian Institute of Sport since the latter part of 1984 has given me contact with

Sports Massage and stretching

many athletes from a wide range of sports, including track and field, swimming, waterpolo, weightlifting, tennis, gymnastics, rowing, basketball, netball, cricket, cycling, hockey and soccer. From years of treating commonly occurring injuries under the guidance of the doctors and physiotherapists at the Institute, I have developed massage treatments which have proved extremely effective.

By slightly modifying my methods, I have developed a program which has enabled athletes to apply massage to themselves, with extremely beneficial results.

The benefits of self-massage are numerous. Unfortunately, the desired massage treatments are not always readily available to the average sportsperson. But knowledge of, and confidence with, self-massage will enable you to treat yourself whenever and wherever it is necessary.

Regular massage treatment often means spending time travelling to appointments and can cost anything from $25 to $50 an hour. Few private health insurance companies recognise massage as a treatment for which fees can be claimed. Self-massage is therefore both inexpensive and time-effective.

Professional masseurs need not fear that people practising self-massage will put them out of business; one of the most positive results of self-massage is that athletes become more aware of their bodies and realise that areas of soft tissue tightness and discomfort can often be relieved by properly administered massage. Take the case of the Australian men's basketball team, which finished fourth at the Seoul Olympic Games.

From previous experience, all members of the team were very much aware that towards the end of a tough tournament the strain of competition would manifest itself in the form of numerous soft tissue aches and pains, as well as general fatigue, which could seriously affect their performance, particularly as proceedings reached a climax.

The players were all instructed in self-massage, with particular emphasis on areas of the body where greatest stress was likely to be felt.

During the Olympic contest, their coach, Dr Adrian Hurley, got them to carry out self-massage daily and as the tournament progressed he observed that more of them than ever before began to seek treatment from the masseurs of the Olympic medical team.

They had come to realise that massage offered relief from the strain of this toughest of all competitions and so sought the assistance of the experts accompanying the Australian Olympic Team in order to maximise the benefits.

This book aims to teach the reader greater awareness of his or her own body and demonstrate, through the use of appropriate stretching and self-massage techniques, that the risk of injury and its adverse effects on performance can be kept to an absolute minimum.

BACKGROUND TO MASSAGE

History of Massage

Human beings have probably always been aware of the wonderful powers of touch — whether for soothing purposes as a mother might stroke the head of her crying infant, for healing, or simply to relieve pain by instinctively rubbing an area which is causing discomfort.

Thousands of years ago massage was an art amongst the Japanese and Chinese, who clearly realised the benefits it had to offer.

Around 3000 BC the Chinese wrote the earliest known books on massage, but it was not until the 18th Century that this information reached Europe when French scholars translated these Oriental classics, providing a foundation from which modern European massage systems were developed.

Like the Japanese and Chinese, the Ancient Romans and Greeks used massage and exercise, combining them with regular baths and exposure to air and sunlight as a means of promoting good health. About 1000 BC, Homer described in the *Odyssey* how beautiful women rubbed and anointed war-worn heroes to rest and refresh them.

In a time when very little was known about human physiology and anatomy, extremely accurate observations of the techniques and effects of massage were made by the Greeks and Romans, indicating that it must have been used extensively and considered to be highly beneficial in the treatment of many conditions.

Hippocrates (460-380 BC) wrote that 'a physician must be experienced in many things, but assuredly also in rubbing', which he called 'anatripsis', referring to the action of rubbing upwards but not down. More than 2000 years ago, when the circulatory and lymphatic systems were not understood, it was recognised that a more favourable result could be achieved by massaging in an upward direction, particularly on the limbs.

The Greek physician Galen drew further conclusions about the use of massage for certain conditions. During his years as physician in the College of Gladiators Galen started work on his most significant contribution to medicine relating to the physiology of the nervous system.

Massage was used extensively at the College of Gladiators and Galen wrote: 'I direct that the strokes and circuits of the hand should be made of many sorts in order that as far as possible all the muscle fibres should be rubbed in every direction.' This suggests that even 1700 years ago practitioners were aware of the benefits of working the soft tissues, not purely in an upwards or transverse direction, but in every direction. This is a practice which has been adopted only in recent times and with some reluctance, but is proving to be very beneficial.

An amusing tale about the Emperor Hadrian, who died in 138 AD, relates how one man derived great advantage from self-massage, while others were not so lucky. Upon entering the public baths one day, the Emperor saw an old soldier rubbing himself against a marble structure. When Hadrian asked him why he did so the old soldier replied, 'Because I have no slave to rub me'. The Emperor took pity on him and gave him two slaves and the funds with which to keep them.

When he next visited the baths Hadrian was greeted by a number of old men, all rubbing themselves vigorously against the marble. But Hadrian was wise to their intent and much to the dissatisfaction of the old men commanded them to rub each other.

During the Dark Ages following the fall of the Roman Empire it seems that the use of massage for healing purposes fell from favour and that knowledge of its techniques survived only because of dedicated monks who preserved the classical texts on the subject.

For most of this time however, Asian societies, particularly China and Japan, continued refining their skills and knowledge, which perhaps helps explain their brilliant methods today. It was not until the Renaissance that massage slowly regained its popularity in Europe.

The Swedish system of massage was introduced by Per Henrick Ling (1776–1839). Ling's approach to massage and his classification of treatments was rapidly adopted in many countries throughout Europe and is still taught in many massage schools today.

Several masseurs have been associated with prominent historical figures. The renowned French surgeon Ambroise Pare (1517–1590) is said to have won favour with a number of French kings by using massage as an integral part of his treatments. More recently, the Finnish masseur Felix Kersten was masseur to Heinrich Himmler and used his influence to save many people from the Nazi terror. Himmler who could only find relief from physical and psychological tension through Kersten's expert treatment, said of him: 'Kersten massages a life out of me with every rub'.

In the late 19th and early 20th centuries there were efforts in Great Britain to re-establish massage as a respectable profession. By the early 1930s the Chartered Society of Massage and Medical Gymnastics numbered over 12,000 registered masseurs and masseuses working all over the United Kingdom.

For much of the past twenty or thirty years it appears that the emphasis on the manual manipulation of the soft tissues has been discarded in favour of more modern types of treatment, including medications and the use of ever-increasing numbers of electrical modalities.

One of the most exciting aspects of medicine and especially sports medicine today is the resurgence of interest in the use of massage. Many excellent schools of massage have been established and are producing graduates with the skills and knowledge worthy of their profession.

Specialists in many fields including doctors, physiotherapists, chiropractors, osteopaths, podiatrists and masseurs are now working closely together. As this co-operation grows and scientific research expands, massage will play an increasingly important role in medicine itself and in the community generally.

The role of Massage in Sports Medicine

Massage is rapidly acquiring a higher profile in sports medicine. It is being used by ever-growing numbers of sportspeople ranging from the top-class athlete to the social jogger.

There are five interrelated ways in which massage can help in body care and fitness. They are:

1. Recovery

Massage considerably accelerates the body's natural healing and recovery processes and is especially beneficial for athletes involved in heavy training and competition.

During training, recovery massage is applied using deep, firm strokes to the length of the muscle. Then, during competition, the massage is lighter with specific attention shown to areas of soreness.

Finally, to facilitate quicker recovery following heavy workouts, you should try to combine self-massage with stretching, concentrating your efforts on the muscle groups most stressed in the preceding session.

Stretching at this time will be most effective if performed soon after the massage, before the muscles have cooled.

Other useful recovery practices include alternative low-level exercise, sauna, spa and flotation therapy.

The Soviet sports scientist Talyshev and some of his colleagues have come up with some important advice on the best times to carry out recovery procedures, particularly as regards morning and evening workouts. Talyshev contends that the quickest way of regaining full 'work capacity' is to begin recovery measures immediately after workouts. But if it is necessary to be back in top gear the following day, he believes it is better to delay such procedures until six or nine hours after the workout or competition. If this activity ends in the evening, then the recuperative program should not be started until the next morning.

2. Prevention

Injury is perhaps the greatest factor preventing you from reaching your real potential. A major injury can stop you engaging in normal activity or even bring your career to a premature end, while a minor one will prevent you from training or performing at full capacity until it clears up.

Regular massage treatments aimed at keeping muscles at their optimal resting length can lower the risk of many soft-tissue and associated overuse injuries. Preventative massage is very thorough and the therapist will use deep, probing strokes to feel for abnormalities in the soft tissues, such as areas of specific muscle tightness. The therapist will also be receptive to your responses, especially any involuntary reactions to pain when palpating tendons and ligaments.

The benefits of massage are cumulative. Over time the conditions of the athlete's soft tissues will continue to improve and this improvement can be maintained with progressively fewer treatments.

People respond differently to deep massage. Some will come out of a session feeling lethargic and some invigorated, while others will feel little immediate change at all. But as the condition of the soft tissues steadily improves over the next twenty-four hours, they will all experience a greater sense of physical wellbeing.

Early recognition of potential problems and the prompt and appropriate application of self-massage and stretching will minimise time out with injury. A preparedness to make self-massage and stretching a part of your daily routine can help to prevent injury altogether.

3. Treatment of Injuries

Many of the more common injuries requiring treatment are associated with the soft tissues and respond well to massage.

In treating injuries by massage it is necessary to have a

sound understanding of anatomy and physiology and to be aware of the contraindications of massage.

Outstanding results are being achieved in the treatment and rehabilitation of many injuries at places like the Australian Institute of Sport where masseurs work in close association with doctors and physiotherapists.

Massage used in treating injuries tends to be more specific in its application, while the techniques used in a single treatment may be quite diverse.

When working a specific area, the therapist must of course seek the patient's advice in ascertaining the exact point needing treatment and deciding on the relative intensity of the massage required. While some treatments may result in considerable discomfort, whether or not pain results should never be the determining factor in massage therapy. Instead, the therapist should rely on his own tactile senses, knowledge, judgement and the patient's responses.

Recent research into the success of massage in treating sporting injuries indicates that significant results can be achieved from short periods of treatment.

You can assist in the treatment of your own injuries by applying massage to appropriate areas, particularly when you are unable to receive treatment from your medical practitioner as regularly as you would like.

It is essential first of all, however, to be sure that self-massage is the right way to deal with a particular injury. You should therefore always consult a doctor or physiotherapist before attempting to treat an injury yourself.

4. Preparation

Massage offers both physiological and psychological benefits when administered immediately before competition.

Psychologically, it will put you in a more positive mood,

reduce tension and mental fatigue, and give you a renewed sense of vigour.

Physically, its effects are even more significant. Pre-competition massage can reduce the pain associated with injury and create greater joint mobility and muscle flexibility.

It's important not to feel too relaxed before a competitive event. The methods used are light and stimulating, often including vibratory techniques and stretching

Some people prefer to have a light massage before warming up while others reverse the order. But either way massage should be an adjunct to the normal warm-up rather than a substitute.

When there is no masseur available before an event or game, self-massage should be employed, particularly if normal warm-up procedures have not produced the desired state of readiness. Stubborn areas of muscle tightness and many soft-tissue injuries will benefit from short sessions of self-massage beforehand.

5. Relaxation

Intensive training, competition, long travel and other such factors can add considerably to normal stress and lead to sub-standard performances. Relaxation massage is one of the best ways of easing the strain.

You should seek relaxation massage when there has been some disruption to your normal sleeping patterns, perhaps as a result of lengthy travel or if you have difficulty coping with competition stress. Relaxation techniques may also be employed immediately before the event if you find yourself over-stimulated, as this may be detrimental to performance.

Relaxation massage is usually administered while the patient is lying in a comfortable, prone position. The techniques used are very soothing and usually cover large areas of the body in a rhythmical fashion, often concentrating on the muscles of the neck, shoulders and back most susceptible to tension from stress and anxiety.

Relaxation massage is the only form of treatment which one cannot perform satisfactorily on oneself. The disjointed nature of the techniques and the fact that they require full personal concentration and effort mean that they have to be applied by somebody else. Generally however, a single treatment is sufficient to produce the desired results.

Contraindications for Massage

In order to avoid the risk of further injury and soft-tissue damage, you should be aware of the circumstances under which the application of massage could be detrimental. If you have the slightest doubt about the appropriateness of massage treatment, you should avoid it until it has been approved by a qualified doctor.

The most significant contraindication of massage comes in its application in the first 48–72 hours following acute soft-tissue trauma. Massage applied to recently traumatised tissue will increase local blood supply and capillary permeability causing even more bleeding into the tissue spaces, further traumatise already damaged cells and result in a larger inflammatory response.

One school of thought still persists in believing that newly damaged or 'corked' muscle tissue can be fixed by immediate 'rubbing' but this can have disastrous consequences.

Occasionally complications can occur to soft-tissue injuries, such as *myositis ossificans*. This condition may follow a direct blow which damages the fibrous connective tissue covering the bone called the periosteum. Bone-forming cells are released into the damaged tissue and form bone plaques. Interference, including massage, may further traumatise the tissue and possibly worsen the condition.

Extended rest and appropriate post-injury care are

essential to cure *myositis ossificans* in view of its
potential dangers.

Massage should never be applied directly over varicose
veins. Their structure is unstable and the pressure
and mechanical action of massage could further damage
them and cause unnecessary complications.

A doctor should be consulted regarding any unusual
eruptions of the skin and massage should not be applied
to affected areas unless medical approval has been given.

A condition known as folliculitis frequently occurs on
areas of the skin where insufficient lubrication has been
used in performing massage. Hair follicles are pulled and
irritated, allowing bacteria to invade the pores of the skin,
resulting in the appearance of small red and often
pus-filled eruptions. These eruptions can be quite painful
and further massage to the area should be avoided until
the condition is controlled. An anti-bacterial skin wash sold
by pharmacists can be used both to clear up and prevent
this irritating condition. In severe cases it may be
necessary to consult a doctor.

Many athletes choose to keep their legs shaved in order
to prevent such irritating skin conditions and avoid the
occasional discomfort resulting from the massage of
particularly hairy limbs.

Direct massage of areas above the lymph glands should
be avoided, particularly when they are swollen and painful
to touch. Lymph glands act as filters and contain
lymphocytes which produce antibodies and are responsible
for the destruction of bacteria and other foreign bodies
that may have invaded the tissues and been drained into
the lymphatic vessels. Massage may inhibit their proper
functioning.

Similarly, it should not be applied to areas of general
tissue swelling, or oedema, as the inflammatory response
may be the result of a particular pathology requiring
specific medical attention, which should be sought
immediately, especially if the disorder has resulted from
known soft-tissue trauma. Only when it has been
thoroughly corrected should massage treatment be
resumed.

Preparing for massage

Effective self-massage requires a degree of personal effort and concentration. Most people will at some time have casually massaged areas of muscle tightness. But this will have been of only minimal benefit. A few simple steps, however, bring better results.

Firstly, allow yourself sufficient time to administer each treatment. The effectiveness of many of the techniques depends upon the repetitiveness of the prescribed strokes. You should only stop when you feel you have done enough, not because you have run out of time. Make sure also that nothing will distract you from satisfactorily completing a treatment.

It is most important that you feel comfortable, sitting with your back against a wall or a piece of furniture. It's a good activity to engage in while watching television.

Oils

Most massage techiques require some form of lubricant which is applied to the skin and allows your hands to slide easily over the area being massaged.

There are many oils suitable for use. Any vegetable oils, including peanut, sunflower, olive and blended oil, will provide sufficient lubrication. Vegetable oils have the advantage of not being readily absorbed into the skin and therefore usually only require a single application. They are also viscous enough to prevent most irritation to the hair follicles. Their disadvantages include the fact that they tend to leave stains on clothing and have a rather unpleasant odour.

Baby oil is popular because it has similar qualities of viscosity and is not readily absorbed into the skin. It is a little more expensive. Other paraffin-based oils such as mineral oil have much the same properties as baby oil and are usually somewhat cheaper.

A wide variety of aromatic oils is available from various health stores, many of which contain certain herbal extracts that are considered to have healing properties.

For massaging a small specific area, any of a number of skin creams can be used. As most creams are absorbed into the skin, they may require several applications during a treatment, but this is not a great problem for only a small area.

Some basic points about self-massage

- Be certain that self-massage is appropriate before commencing treatment. If in doubt, get medical advice first.
- Begin each massage using light strokes. This allows you to assess the condition of your soft tissues and identify areas of tenderness. Initial light stroking also allows your soft tissues time to respond favourably to massage.
- Gradually increase the pressure of your strokes as the massage proceeds. Guided by your personal tolerance of pain, your strokes should steadily become more probing in order to affect deeper muscle tissue. Loosening up tight muscles will not always be a pleasant experience. But any discomfort should still feel as though it's doing the muscle good without causing damage. If it's too painful use a lighter pressure and make the treatments more frequent.
- Use as much of the full hand as possible on the areas. This will enable you to vary the pressure and give you greater control over each stroke.
- Stretch after each massage. Your muscles will be warm from increased blood-flow, letting you get maximum benefit from stretching. Use the stretch-relaxation method and conclude each stretching sequence with a static hold of approximately thirty seconds.
- Seek appropriate medical advice if the condition you're treating shows no improvement after two or three properly conducted self-massage sessions.

Technical Terms

- Anterior   Nearer to or at the front of the body.
- Deep (internal)   Away from the surface of the body.
- Distal   Situated away from the point of origin of a limb or a bone.
- Inferior   Away from the head or toward the lower part of a structure; generally refers to structures in the trunk.
- Lateral   Further from the midline of the body or a structure.
- Medial   Nearer the midline of the body or a structure.
- Parietal   Pertaining to the outer wall of a body cavity.
- Posterior   Nearer to or at the back of the body.
- Prone   Lying face downwards.
- Proximal   Nearer the attachment of an extremity to the trunk or a structure.
- Superficial   Toward the surface of the body.
- Superior   Toward the head or upper part of a structure; generally refers to structures in the trunk.
- Supine   Lying on the back.

MASSAGE TECHNIQUES

Muscles of the anterior and lateral compartments of the lower leg

1.

Sit on the floor with the leg to be massaged bent to an angle of approximately 45°.

Press the flattened pads of both thumbs into the muscle slightly inferior to the knee and lateral to the tibia. The hands, with fingers slightly spread, should be lightly wrapped around the leg. Select an appropriate pressure and maintain it as you push your thumbs from your knee, downwards to a point just superior to your ankle. (Fig. 1a)

At the completion of each stroke slide your hands lightly over the skin back to the starting position.

During the initial strokes the thumbs will be guided by the lateral border of the tibia. As the massage progresses the strokes are moved laterally from the tibia, until the entire surface area of the anterior and lateral compartments has been thoroughly massaged.

You will find the lateral compartment easier to reach if you allow your knee to drop slightly inwards.

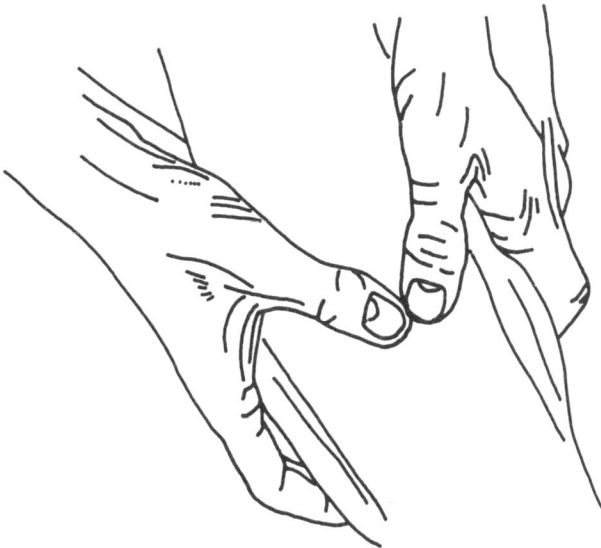

Fig. 1a

2.

The second technique for the anterior and lateral compartments of the lower leg also begins with the leg to be massaged bent to an angle of approximately 45°.

Press the flattened pads of both thumbs into the muscle slightly superior to the ankle and lateral to the tibia. (Fig. 2a) Concentrate on keeping the thumb-pressure constant as you slowly straighten your leg, keeping your foot in contact with the ground, while at the same time slowly straightening your back. (Fig. 2b)

Fig. 2a

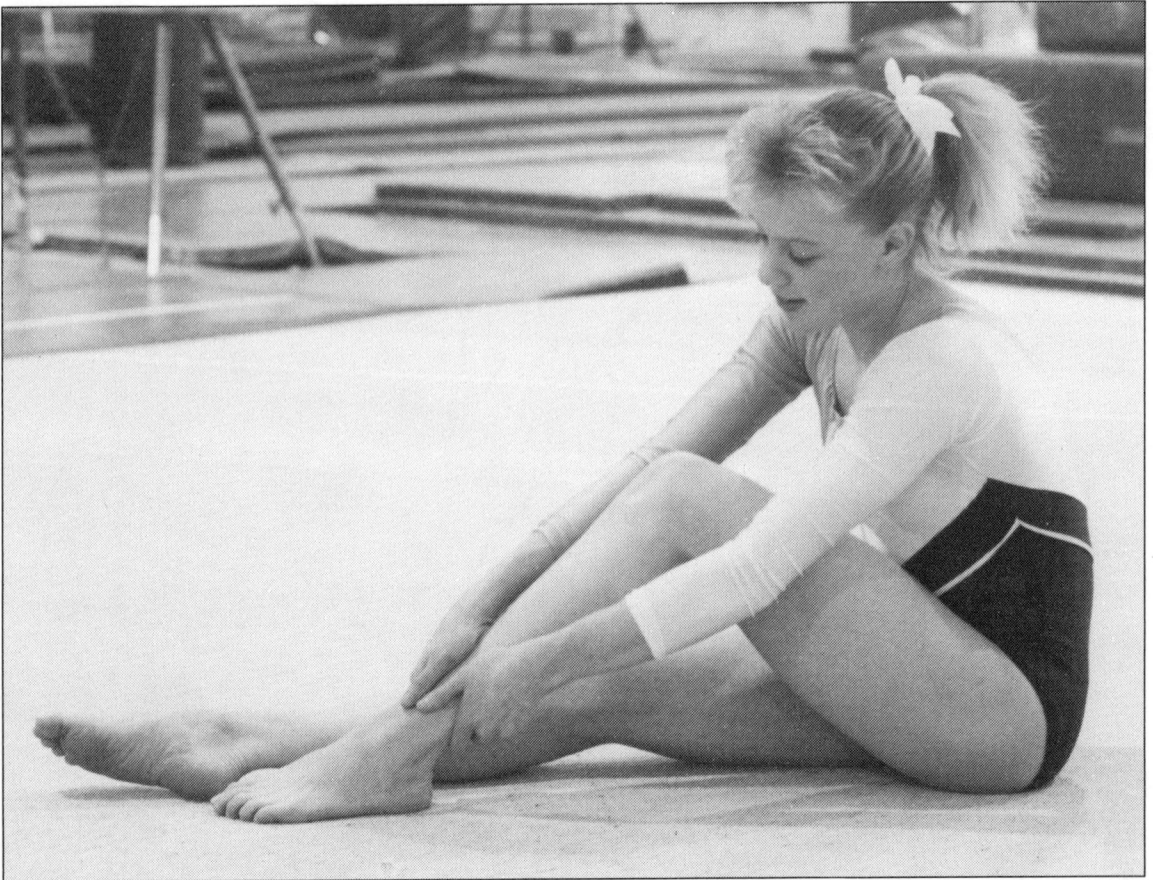

In doing so your hands will be drawn along your leg towards the knee.

This technique will save your arms and shoulders from becoming tired.

Again the strokes progress from the tibia laterally, until the entire surface area of the anterior and lateral compartments has been covered.

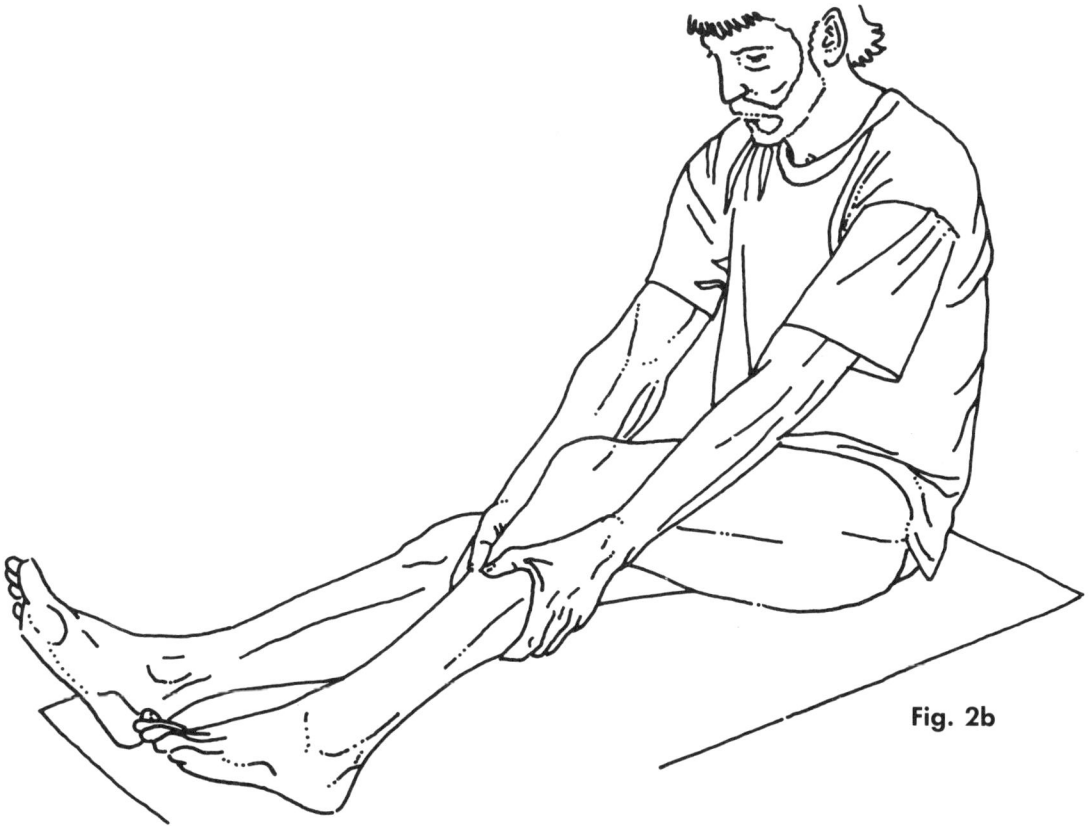

Fig. 2b

Superficial posterior and deep posterior compartments of the lower leg

3.

The first two techniques for the posterior compartments of the lower leg have the same effects. However, some may find one technique easier to perform than the other.

The only real difference in these techniques is the way in which the hands are held.

Technique A uses the fingers of both hands. The fingers are held together and pressed into the muscle while the thumbs rest on top of the leg. (Fig. 3a)

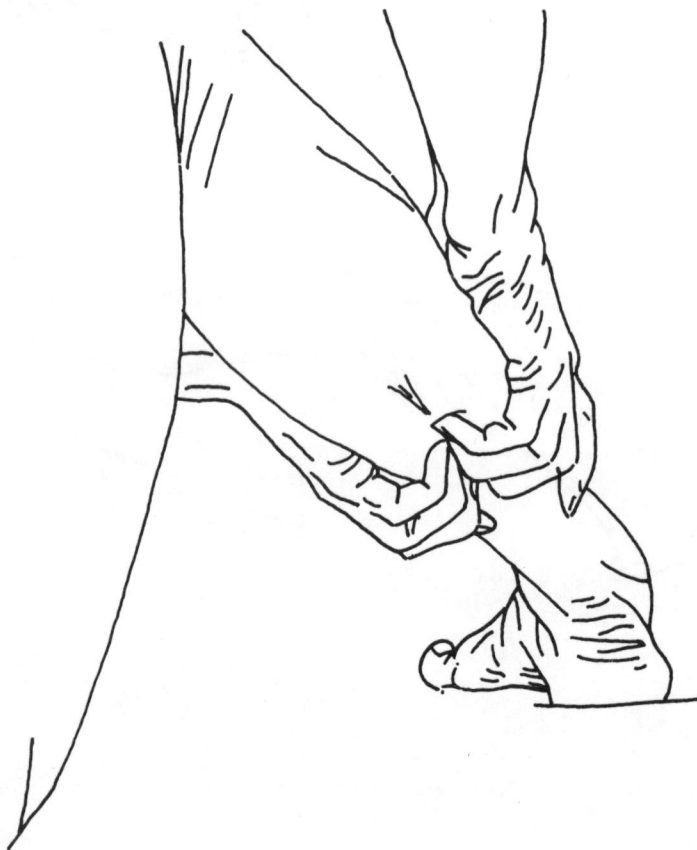

Fig. 3a

Technique B uses the thumbs, which are pressed into the muscle at the back of the leg while the fingers are held on top of the leg. (Fig. 3b)

Both techniques begin at the Achilles tendon and move upwards along the leg to the space behind the knee.

Each stroke is started with the leg bent to an angle of approximately 45° and again the leg and back are simultaneously straightened in order to draw the hands upwards along the leg.

If the knee is bent inwards at the starting position, the medial aspects of the posterior compartments are easy to reach. If the knee is bent outwards at the starting position, the lateral aspects are easily reached.

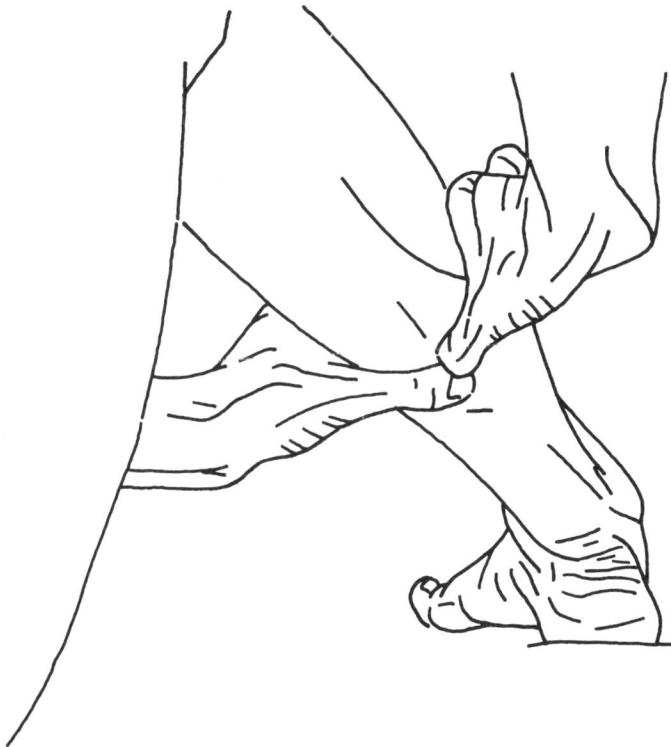

Fig. 3b

4.

The leg to be massaged is bent to an angle of approximately 45° and held slightly outwards, away from the midline of the body.

Press the pads of both thumbs into the muscle slightly superior to the ankle on the medial aspect of the tibia. (Fig. 4)

As the knee and back are straightened the thumbs will be drawn along the leg with each stroke finishing at the knee.

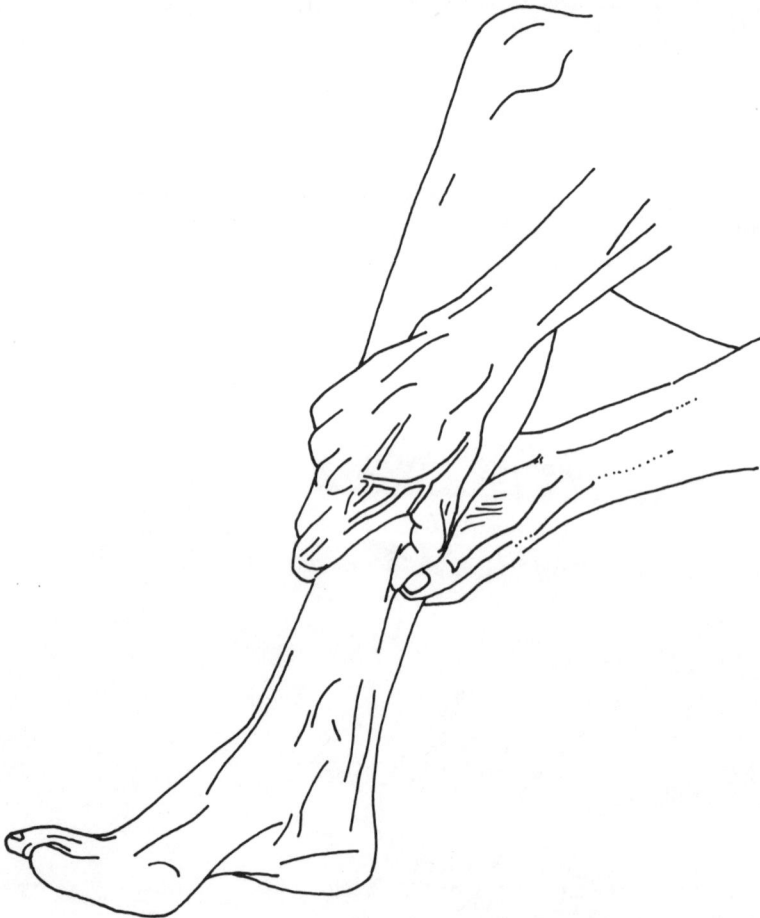

Fig. 4

5.

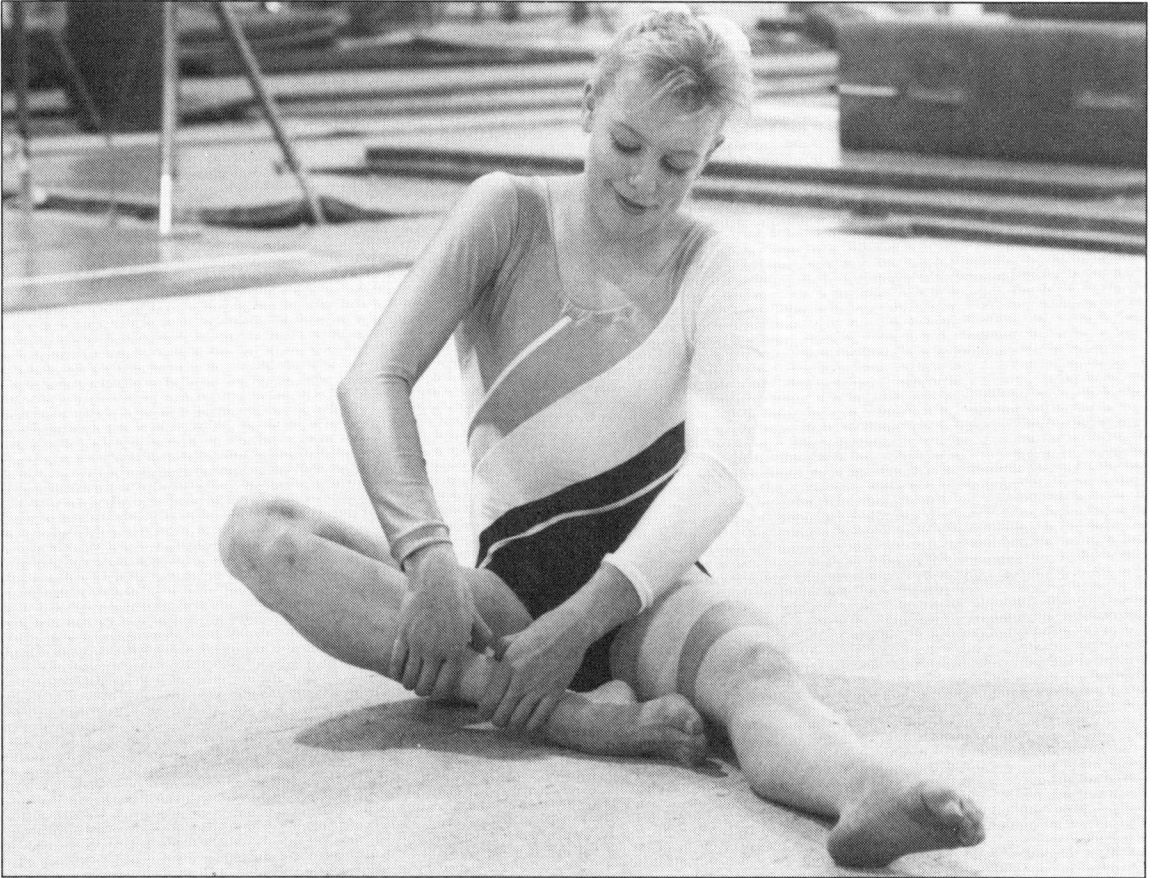

Fig. 5

The final technique for the lower leg is a very strong one and can be used to massage specific areas of tightness along the medial border of the tibia.

Sit on the floor with the foot of the leg to be massaged drawn close to the middle of your body.

Grasp the leg so that the fingers of both hands sit on top of the tibia. Holding your thumbs back to back, press them quite pointedly into the muscle of the medial side of the tibia close to the ankle. Maintain the initial pressure as you move your thumbs in an opposite direction from one another, separating them by no more than 3 cm. If they

23

are further apart pressure will be lost, making the stroke less effective.

Slide the bottom thumb up to meet the top thumb where it has finished. Again press your thumbs into the soft tissue and repeat the stroke. The strokes will overlap and a thorough massage effect will be achieved. (Fig. 5)

When massaging from the ankle to the knee, areas of particular soreness may be found. These areas will inevitably be very tight. Unless they are extremely painful it is advisable to pause over them, repeating the stroke several times before moving on.

These strokes should be made very deliberately and quite slowly. It may take one to two minutes to massage the whole of the lower leg. This may be repeated three to four times.

Quadriceps

6.

The quadricep muscles can be vibrated using lightly clenched fists, which are alternately struck upon the leg with a rapid flicking motion of the wrists.

By rolling the leg inwards the lateral muscles can easily be reached and by rolling the leg outwards the muscles on the medial part of the leg can be vibrated.

It is a good idea to begin massage to the upper legs with two to three minutes of pounding, as it will have a general loosening effect upon the muscle before deeper massage techniques are used.

7.

To massage the lateral side of the quadriceps, including the iliotibial band, hold the middle three fingers of one hand tightly together with the centre finger slightly bent so that the tips of these fingers are almost in line with one another.

Press your other hand on top of the hand which is in contact with your lower leg so as to add greater pressure and control to the stroke. (Fig. 7)

Having established a suitable pressure, maintain it as you push your fingers along the length of your leg to the lateral part of your knee. Release the pressure at the knee and slide your hands back along your leg to the starting position.

Fig. 7

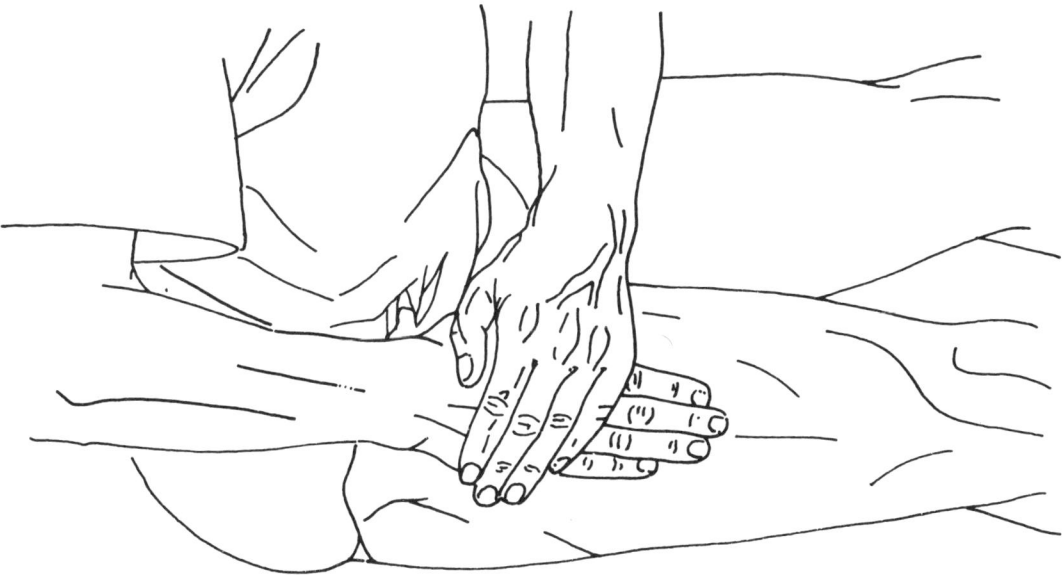

Sports Massage and stretching

8.

Holding your thumbs side by side, press them into the muscle on top of your leg close to the hip. You should allow your fingers to lightly wrap around your leg.

While maintaining a constant pressure, push your thumbs down your leg towards your knee. (Fig. 8)

During the full length of the stroke your thumbs should be held together. If the thumbs separate, pressure will be lost, making the stroke less effective.

The leg can be rolled inwards in order to reach the lateral muscles and rolled outwards to reach the muscles on the medial part of the upper leg.

Fig. 8

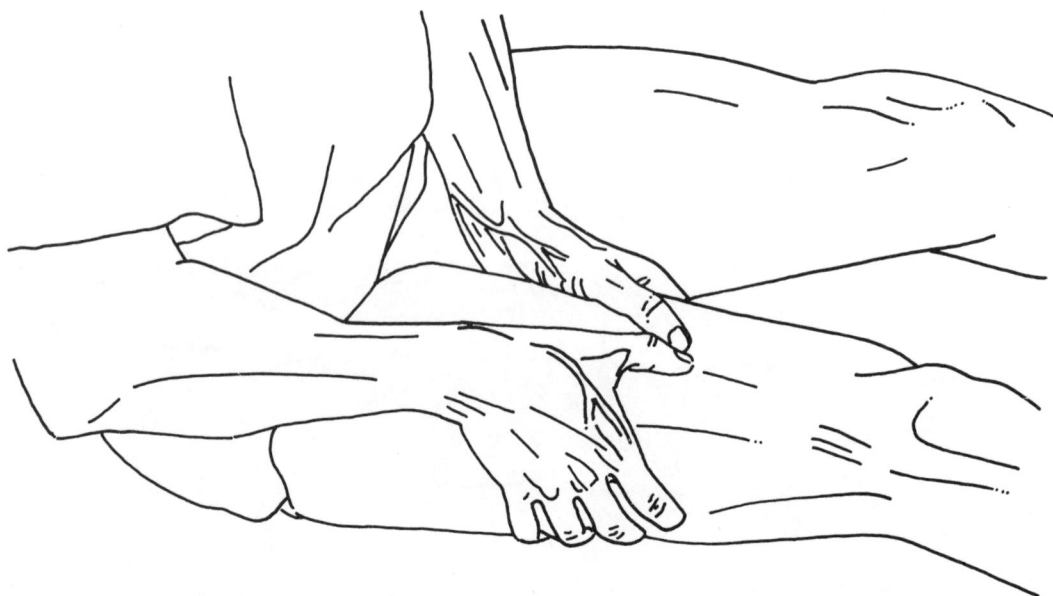

9.

To massage a specific muscle area, place both hands, with fingers slightly spread, on your leg, holding your thumbs over the area to be massaged.

Move the thumbs in a circular fashion, with just one thumb at a time coming into contact with the leg and moving from the point of contact towards the knee. After pushing the first thumb along the muscle for several centimetres, lift it off to allow the other thumb to come into contact with the leg.

While maintaining continuous contact using this alternative thumb motion, your hands can be moved slowly along your leg towards your knee. (Fig. 9)

Fig. 9

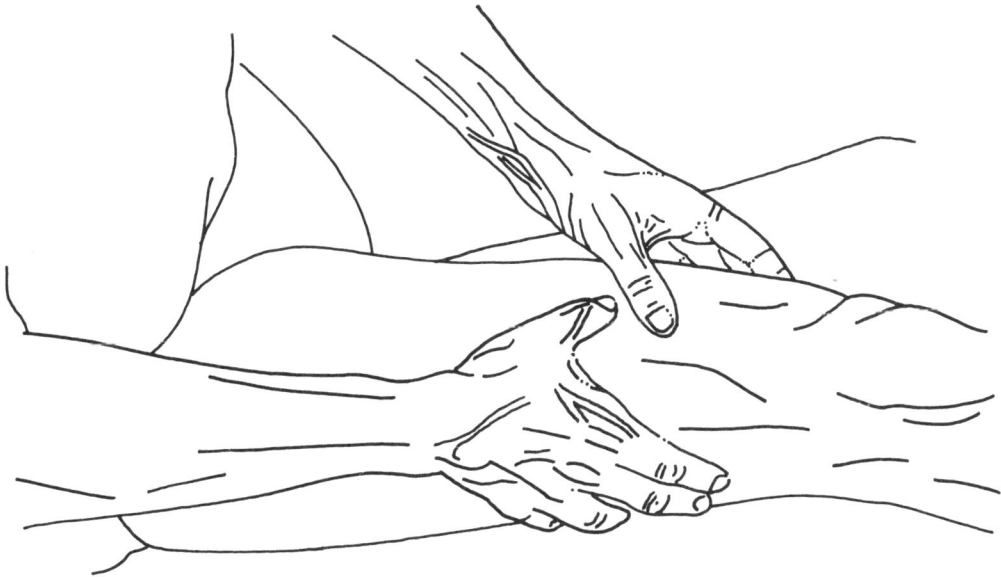

10.

While massaging your legs you may find specific areas of tightness appearing as small lumps or knots. These are often found close to the knee and they may not have seemed to respond a great deal to the previous massage techniques.

A particularly effective technique for loosening out such areas involves pressing the tips of both thumbs firmly into an area of tightness. (Fig. 10) While maintaining the pressure with your thumbs, slowly contract your quadriceps and hold the contraction for several seconds. As you slowly contract your muscles you will feel them collecting under your thumbs and if the area is particularly tight your thumbs will tend to be pushed upwards, out of the muscles.

Fig. 10

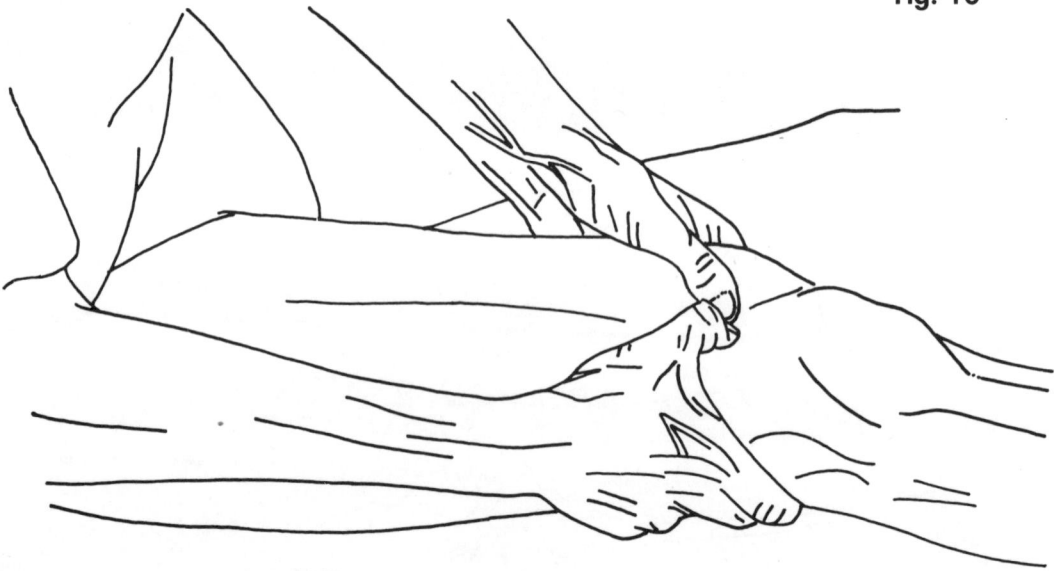

After holding this position for several seconds, slowly relax your muscles and then release your thumb pressure.

Apply this technique to a specific area only three or four times during a massage.

If you find that the entire length of a muscle feels very tight, this technique can be used to work systematically from near the hip all the way down to the knee.

Specific areas of tightness can also be dealt with simply by pressing your thumbs firmly into the muscle and rocking them backwards and forwards for approximately fifteen seconds before repositioning them and repeating the action.

Adductors

11.

The adductors can be massaged in a similar fashion to the lateral part of the quadriceps and the iliotibial band.

Press the tips of the middle fingers of one hand into the muscles on the inside of your leg, close to your groin. Exert additional force by pressing your other hand over the one in contact with your leg. Slowly push your fingers along the inside of your leg until you reach the medial part of your knee. (Fig. 11)

Where specific areas of tightness and pain are felt the thumbs can be pressed into the muscle and rocked gently backwards and forwards.

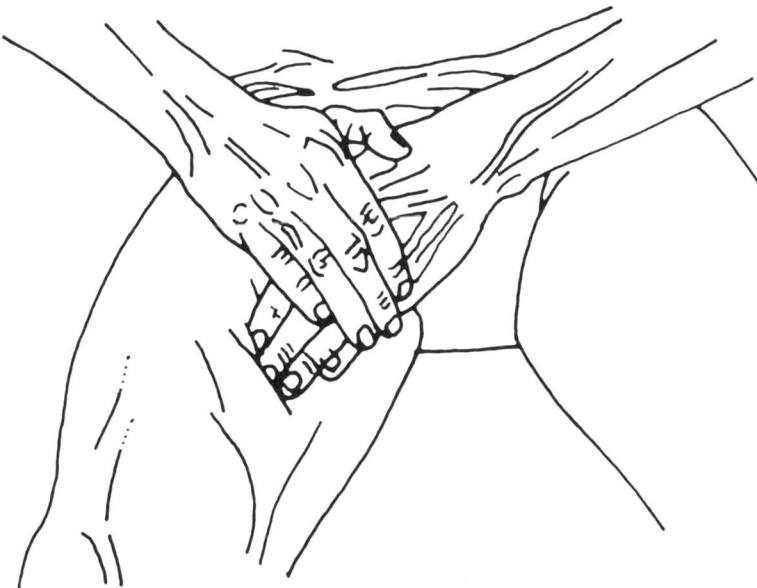

Fig. 11

Summary

There is no strictly correct or incorrect sequence of techniques to use when massaging the quadriceps.

However, an effective self-massage treatment of the quadriceps and adductors would begin with a few minutes of gentle pounding, followed by long strokes moving towards the knee using only a light pressure to begin with and progressing to a relatively firm pressure. The long strokes will generally be followed by more specific techniques that concentrate on particular areas of tightness. These deeper techniques can be interspersed with both light and deep longitudinal strokes.

The massage may then be completed with a few more minutes of gentle pounding.

Hamstrings

12.

To massage the hamstring group of muscles, lie on your back with the leg to be massaged held in a position of hip and knee flexion of approximately 90°. (Fig. 12a)

Holding your fingers together, press the tips of them into your hamstrings so that the backs of your fingers of both hands are in contact with one another. (Fig. 12b) By moving your fingers across the muscles it will be easy to locate areas of tightness.

Press the fingers of both hands firmly into the muscle. While maintaining the pressure, slowly draw your fingers downwards towards the buttocks while at the same time slowly straightening your knee. (Fig. 12c)

This technique will be most effective if an area of only 10–15 cm is massaged with each straightening of the leg.

A second technique which can be used in combination with this involves pressing the fingers firmly into the muscles and rocking backwards and forwards through an area of tightness while the leg is again held in a position of approximately 90° of hip and knee flexion.

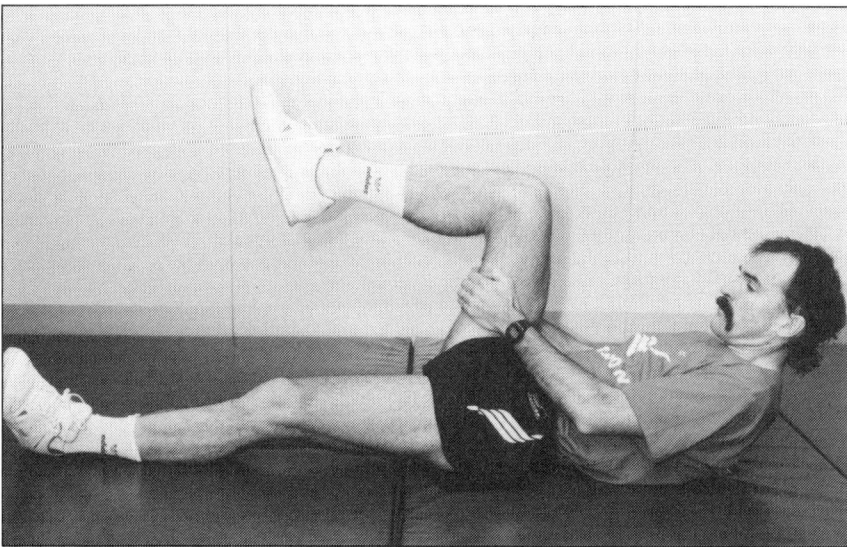

Fig. 12a

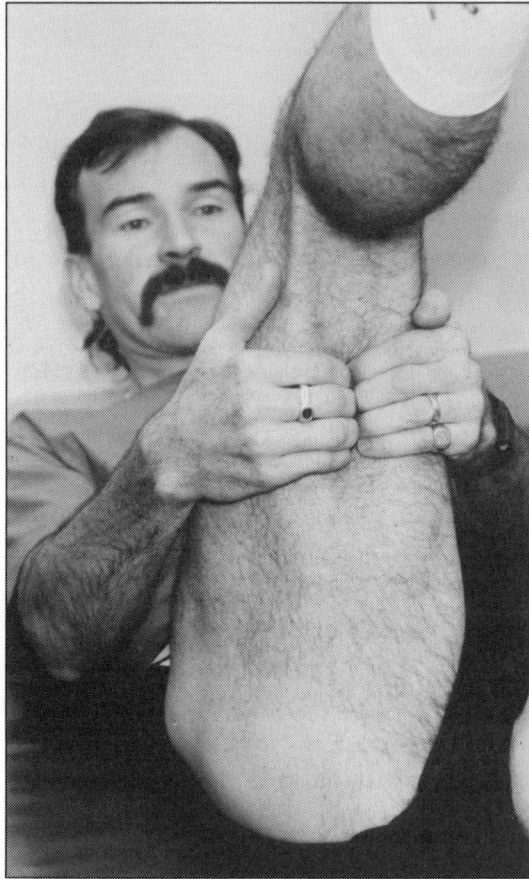

Fig. 12b

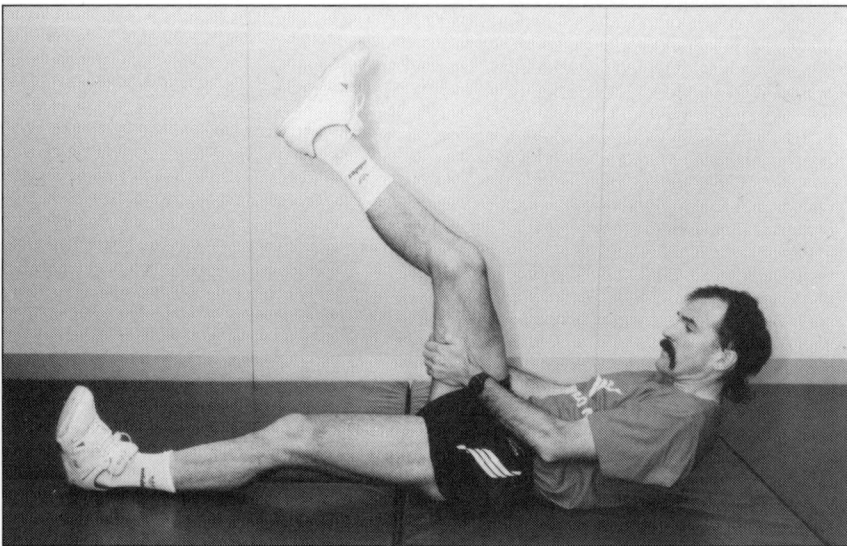

Fig. 12c

Buttocks

13.

The muscles of the buttocks and lower back are, as might be imagined, difficult areas to massage, particularly when you're endeavouring to massage these areas yourself.

A massage technique used by various medical practitioners called palpation involves pressing the tips of the thumbs in a rhythmical downward motion and then releasing them.

Another commonly used technique is that of acupressure, whereby pressure is applied with the thumbs to certain points of the body. This pressure can be applied and maintained for any length of time from several seconds to several minutes.

A simple technique has been developed whereby you can palpate or apply a more constant pressure to muscles of your buttocks and lower back yourself.

Lie on your back and place a golf ball under your buttocks, making sure it's not directly beneath any bony areas. (Fig. 13a)

Fig. 13a

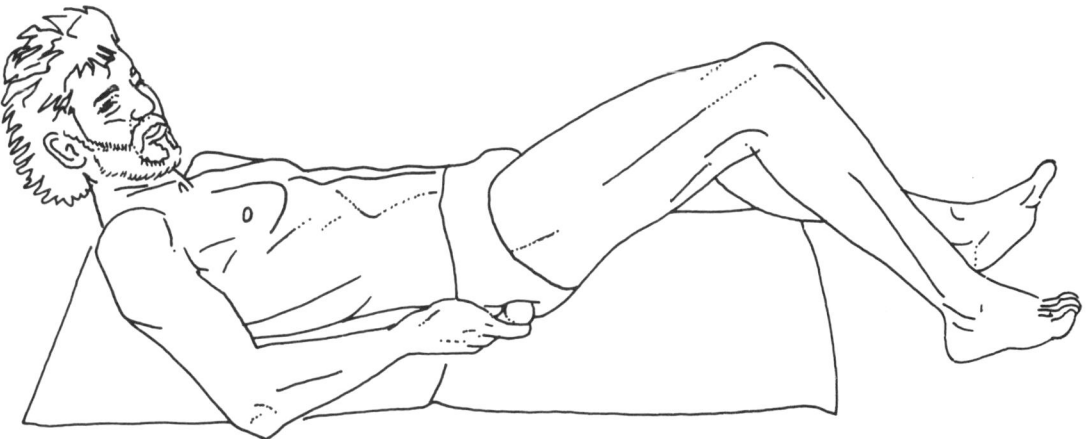

Bend the leg opposite the buttock under which the golf ball has been placed with hip and knee flexion of approximately 45°. (Fig. 13b)

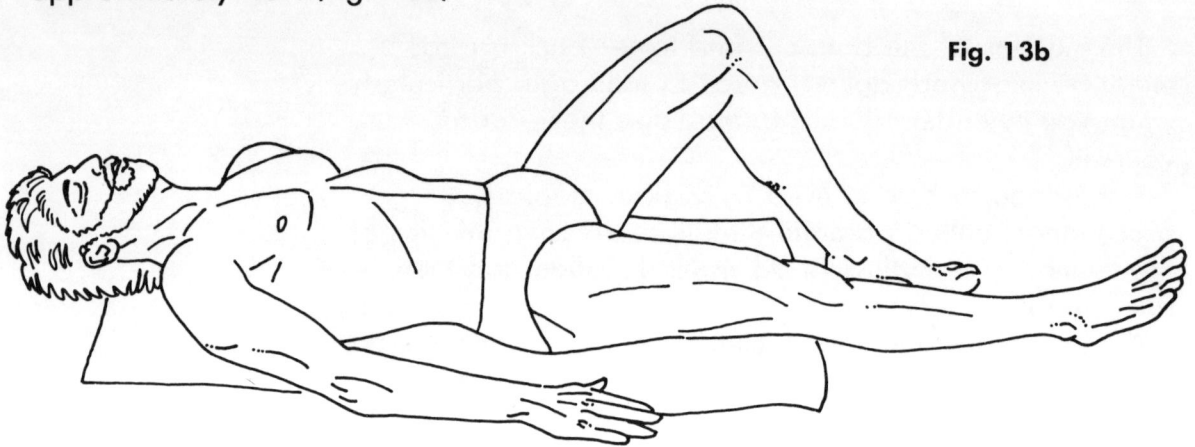

Fig. 13b

Rotate the bent leg across to the opposite side of the body to distribute greater weight over the golf ball, causing the muscles above the ball to press down on it. Maintain the pressure for several seconds and then release it by moving the leg back to its original position. Repeat this action as many times as you feel necessary. Reposition the golf ball and go through the process again. (Fig. 13c)

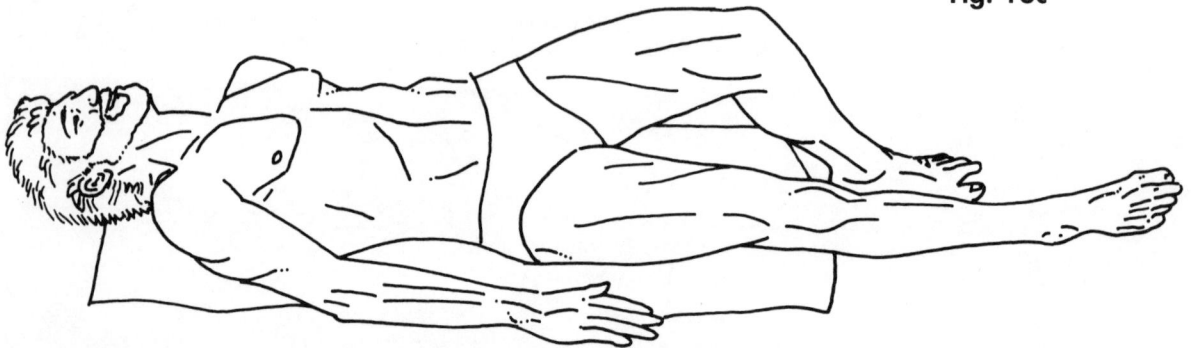

Fig. 13c

Using this technique, the muscles of the buttocks, in particular the gluteus medius and piriformis, can be palpated and a loosening effect achieved.

Lower back

14.

As with the buttocks, a golf ball is required to palpate the muscles of the lower back.

Lying in the supine position place the ball under the area of tightness requiring treatment. As long as you make sure it's not directly beneath any prominent bone structure, because of your natural lumbar curve you will most likely hardly be aware that the ball is there. (Figs. 14a & b)

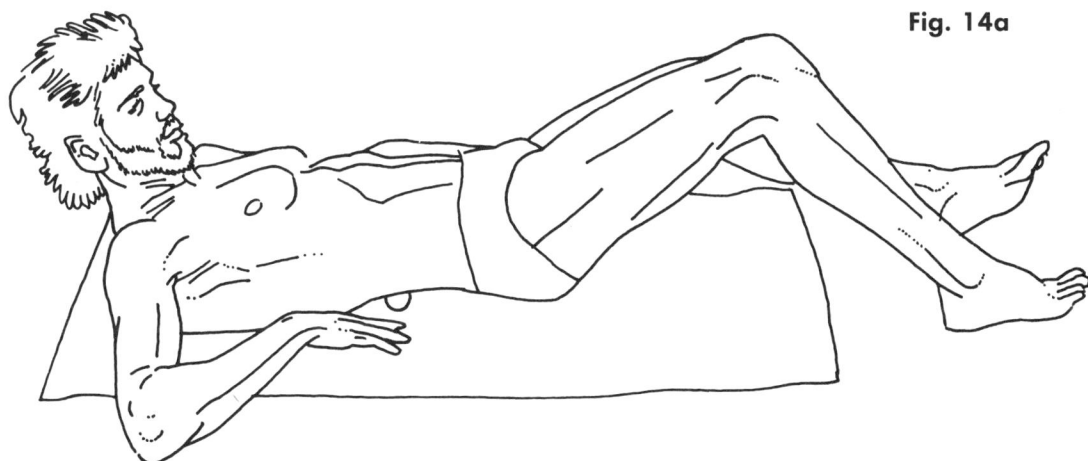

Fig. 14a

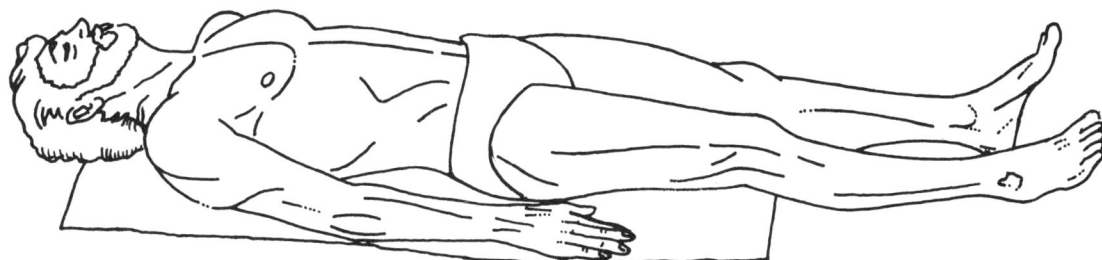

Fig. 14b

Sports Massage and stretching

Work through the following series of movements, adding more pressure to the golf ball until you find a position in which the muscles of the lower back can be satisfactorily palpated.

First, bend your knees slightly, drawing your feet a little closer to your buttocks. Your lower back will be flattened a little and you will feel a greater pressure in the area where the golf ball is situated.

Should you feel this pressure is not sufficient, bend your knees so that your feet are as close to your buttocks as you can get them. Your lower back will now be almost completely flat. (Fig. 14c)

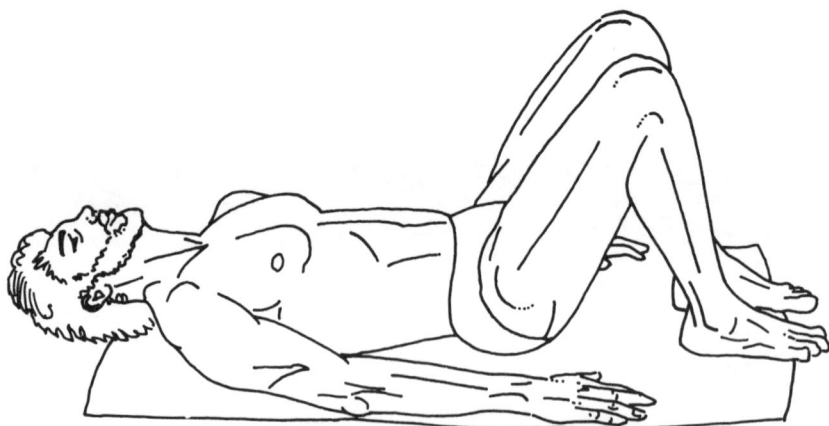

Fig. 14c

If the pressure is still not sufficient, rotate both your legs to the side under which the golf ball is placed. Hold your legs in this rotated position for several seconds. Then remove the pressure by returning your legs to their original position. Repeat this movement as many times as you feel necessary.

Should greater pressure still be required, you can raise your feet by lifting them and holding your legs in a position of hip and knee flexion of 90°. (Fig. 14d) The weight of the legs will now be pressing down on the golf ball, providing what is for most people a very firm pressure. A palpating effect is achieved by simply raising and lowering the legs.

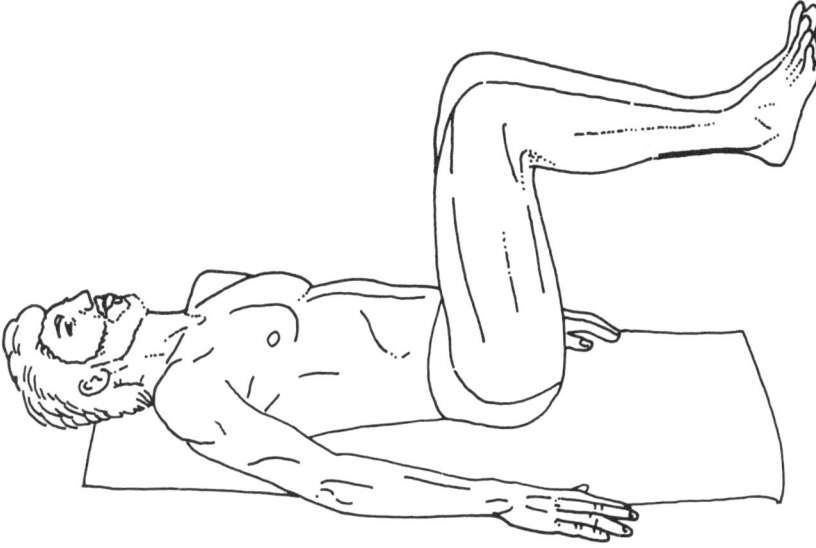

Fig. 14d

The final position involves holding the leg of the same side under which the golf ball is placed close to your chest. Using both hands, pull your knee to your chest while leaving the other leg flat on the ground. (Fig. 14e)

By now you will most likely have found a position for exerting a suitable pressure on the area to be palpated. Move your legs to a position which achieves that pressure, hold it for a few seconds, then return to a position where the pressure is removed.

Repeat the process until the desired effect has been achieved.

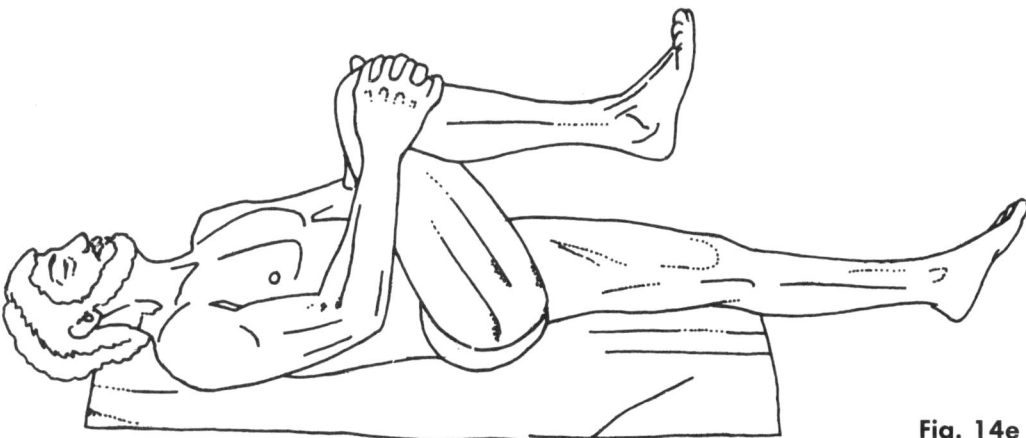

Fig. 14e

15.

Another massage technique for the lower back requires you to stand with your lower back flattened against a wall and your knees slightly bent.

Place a golf ball between the wall and the area of your lower back that you wish to massage.

While applying firm pressure to the ball, repeatedly straighten and bend your legs. As you do this the ball will roll up and down over the area you want massaged.

This technique has a similar effect to a masseur using his thumbs to apply a firm pressure along your muscles.

Middle and upper back

16.

The muscles of the middle and upper back, particularly the erector spine muscles, can be massaged using the same technique.

It is simply a matter of standing with your back to a wall and positioning the golf ball between the area you wish to massage and the wall.

Bend and straighten your legs repeatedly to roll the ball over any areas of tightness.

17.

Many people experience tightness and discomfort in the muscles between the shoulder blades, particularly in the rhomboids and the lower part of the trapezius.

The same technique as prescribed for those of the middle back can be used in combination with stretching to loosen these muscles and relieve associated pain.

It is often preferable to use a firm squash ball as it will mould to the contours of the body and a golf ball may be too hard when this area is particularly tight.

Standing with your knees slightly bent and your upper
back flattened against the wall, place the squash ball
between your vertebrae and scapula. Bend and straighten
your legs repeatedly as you press your back and
shoulders over the ball. (Figs. 17a & b)

A few minutes using this technique, interspersed with
rhomboid stretching techniques, can be very effective in
reducing both pain and tightness.

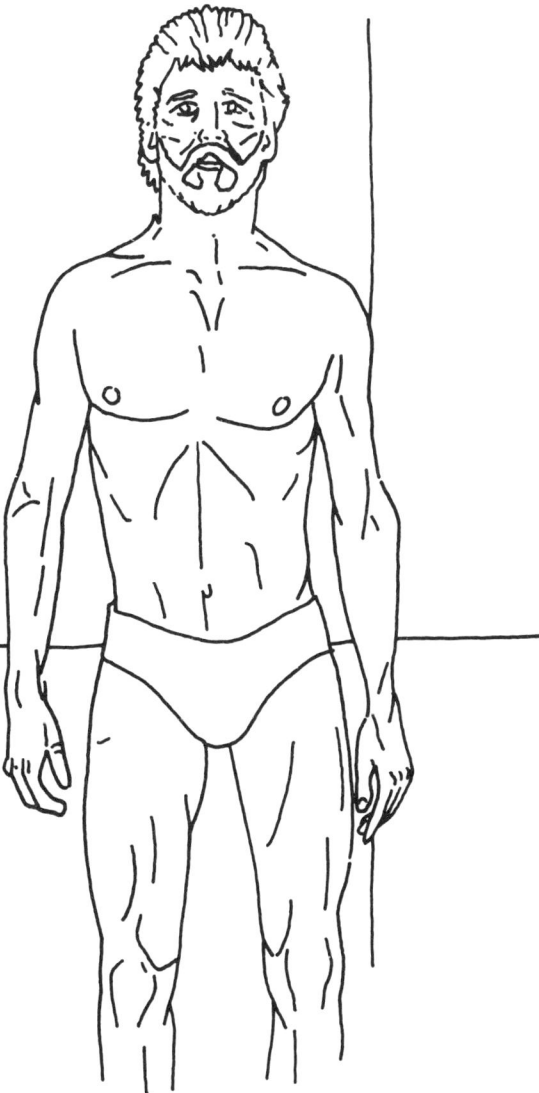

Fig. 17a

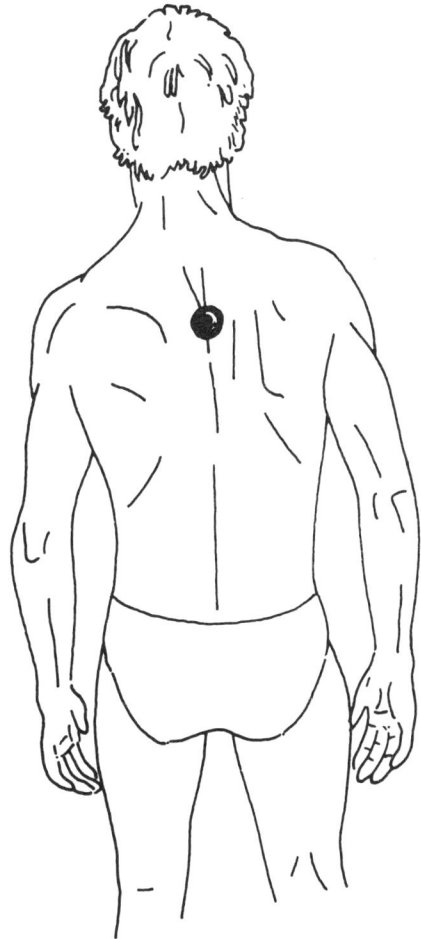

Fig. 17b

Infraspinatus

18.

The infraspinatus can be massaged by standing slightly side-on to the wall and placing a squash ball between the wall and your scapula.

Move your shoulder in a circular fashion so that the ball rolls over the surface of your scapula massaging the infraspinatus. (Fig. 18)

Towards the centre of the infraspinatus muscle there is a very strong pressure-point which can help relieve muscle tightness in this area when massaged. Should you find a point which is particularly tight and sore, apply a downward pressure so that the squash ball presses into it. Hold the pressure for several seconds, then slowly release it and repeat the procedure four or five times.

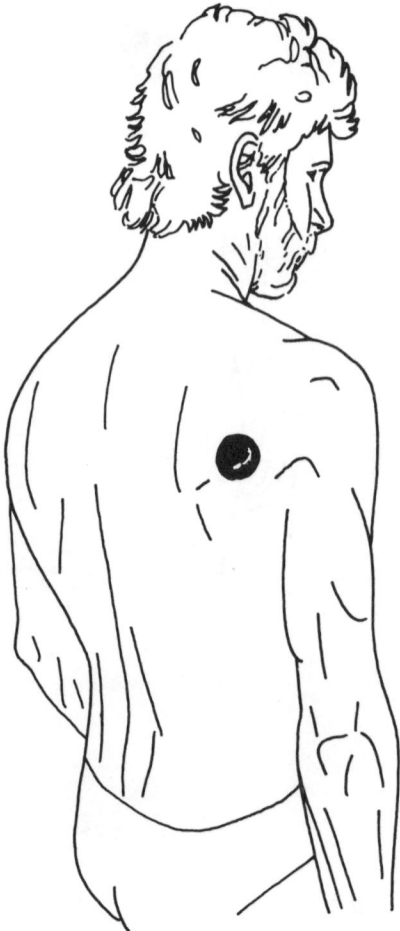

Fig. 18

Trapezius

19.

Much of the trapezius can be massaged by using two techniques.

The first deals with the fibres which originate in the neck and travel down to cover the upper part of the shoulders.

With your head in an upright position, press the pads of your middle three fingers of the hand opposite to the side you are massaging into the muscle towards the back of your neck and slightly below your skull. (Fig. 19a)

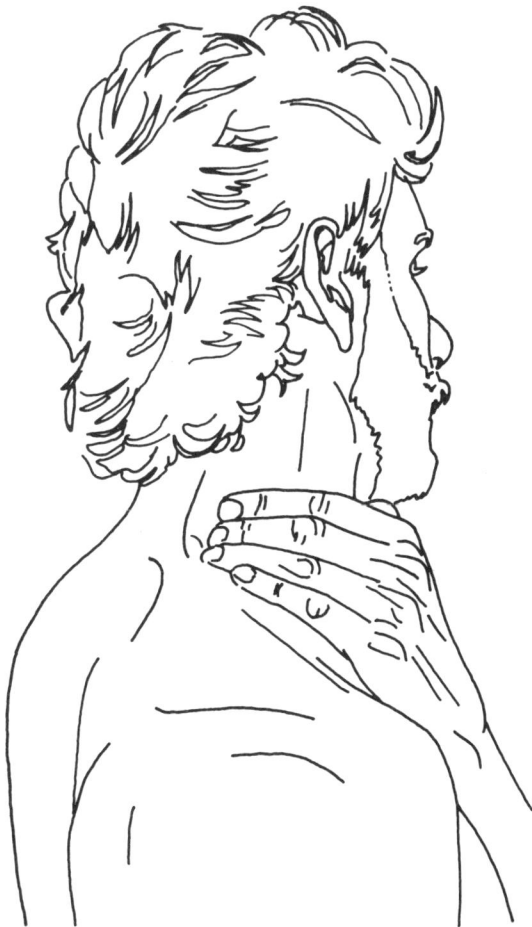

Fig. 19a

Maintaining a constant pressure, which should only be light for the initial strokes, drag your fingers towards your shoulder while at the same time flexing or tilting your head to the opposite side. This will slightly stretch the upper fibres of the trapezius. (Fig. 19b)

As the stroke finishes over the shoulder, return your head to an upright position and repeat. The length of each stroke can be varied with each lateral flexion of the head.

The technique which is used to massage the lower fibres of trapezius that travel down to the twelfth thoracic vertebra is the same as that used to massage the rhomboids and/or the middle back.

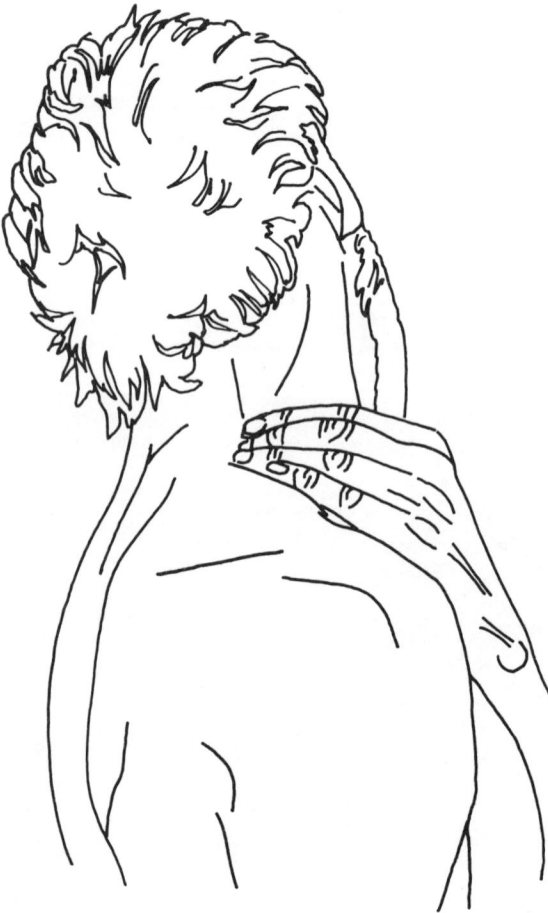

Fig. 19b

Supraspinatus

20.

Because the supraspinatus sits in the supraspinous fossa of the scapula and is covered by the upper fibres of the trapezius as they pass down over the shoulder, it may be necessary to spend a few minutes massaging this region before attempting to effectively massage the supraspinatus.

Press the fingertips of one hand into the muscle at the top of the opposite shoulder, feeling through your trapezius for a tight area of the supraspinatus. Should the supraspinatus be the cause of shoulder pain it will feel tight and sore when palpated. (Fig. 20a)

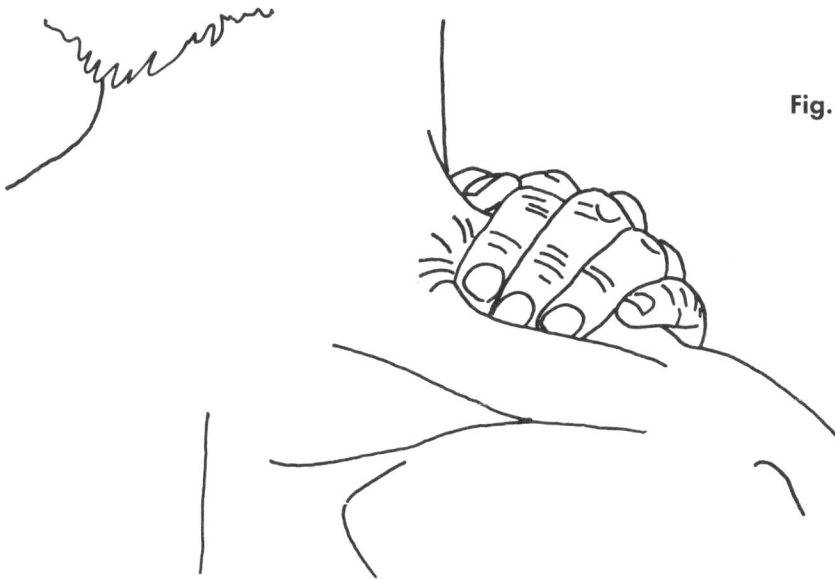

Fig. 20a

Sports Massage and stretching

Press your fingers firmly into the muscle and maintain a constant pressure as you rock your fingers backwards and forwards so as to massage the muscle transversely. Continue for fifteen to twenty seconds, then release the pressure, re-position your fingers and repeat the process. (Fig. 20b)

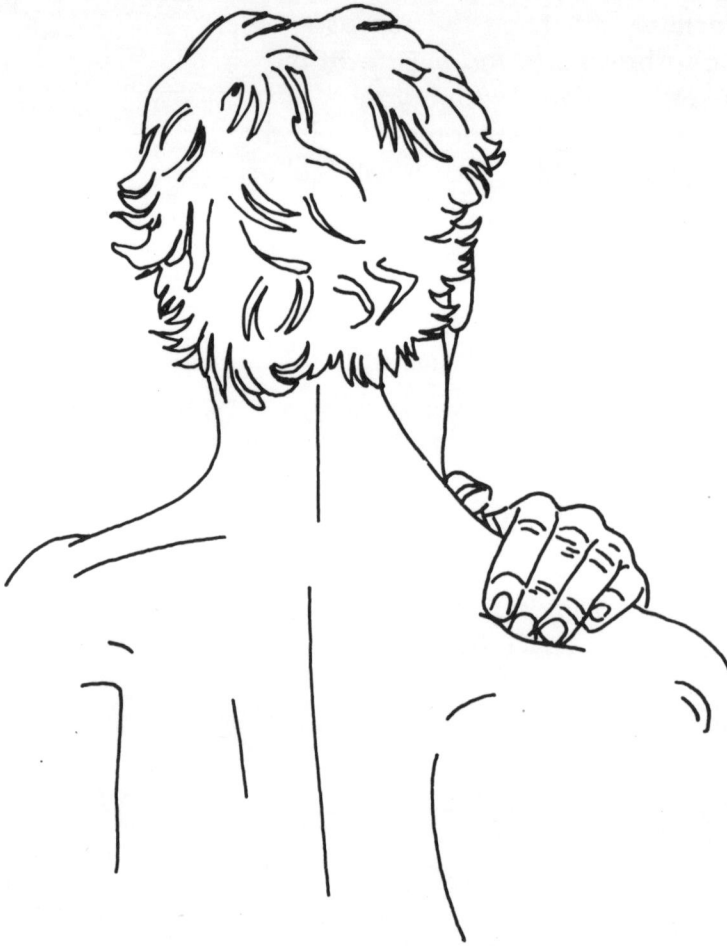

Fig. 20b

This transverse technique is used in combination with long strokes. Press your fingers into the muscle and while maintaining a constant pressure pull your fingers along the length of the muscle, moving either laterally or medially.

44

Latissimus dorsi

21.

Place the hand of the side you wish to massage behind your neck, thus slightly stretching the latissimus dorsi. Use the tips of your fingers to feel transversely for areas of tightness. (Fig. 21a)

Fig. 21a

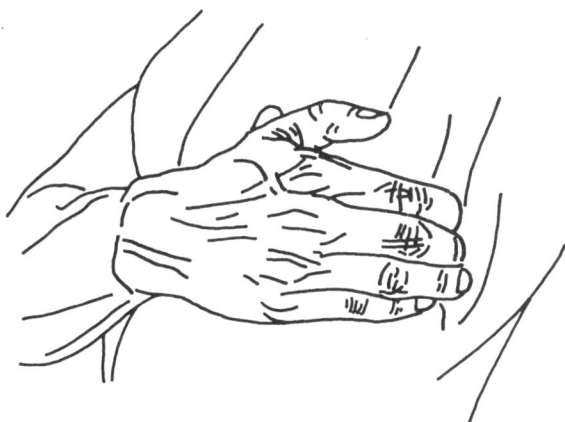

Fig. 21b

Press your fingers firmly into the muscle and while maintaining a constant pressure draw your fingers downwards along the latissimus dorsi. Cover only short areas of approximately 10 cm with each stroke. (Fig. 21b)

A transverse technique can also be used in which the fingers are pressed into an area of tightness and rocked backwards and forwards. Ideally, the two techniques should be carried out alternately.

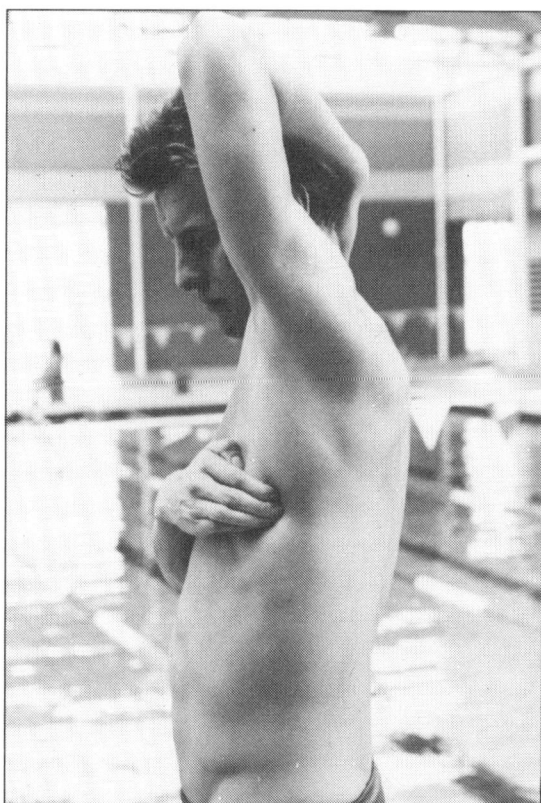

Pectoralis major and minor

22.

Hold the middle three fingers of one hand tightly together with the centre finger slightly bent so that the tips of these fingers are almost in line with each other. (Fig.22a)

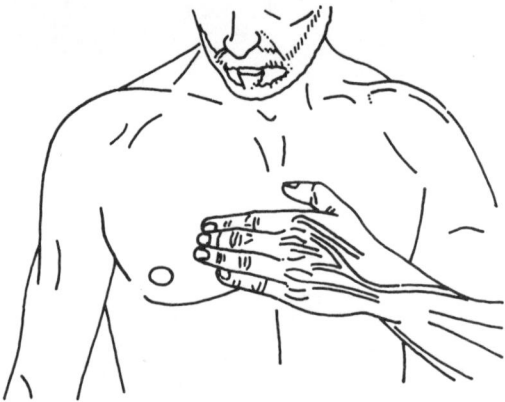

Fig. 22a

Fig. 22b

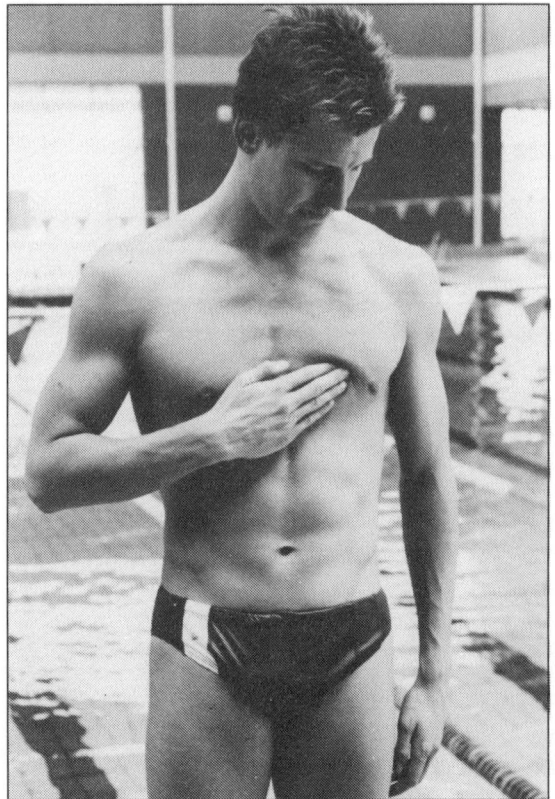

Press the pads of these fingers into the muscle close to your sternum.

Maintain a constant pressure as you push your fingers along the muscle, moving from your sternum to your shoulder. (Fig. 22b)

23.

By placing one hand behind your head your pectoral or breast muscles will be placed on stretch. (Fig. 23)

This will allow you to more effectively massage the musculotendinous junctions and tendons of the muscles.

Again, each stroke begins at the sternum and moves towards your shoulder.

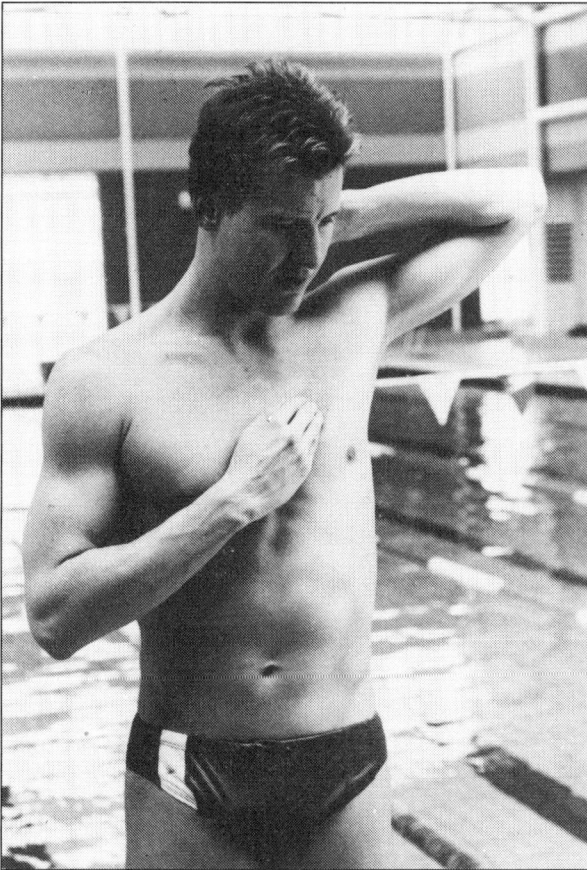

Fig. 23

47

24.

Place one hand behind your neck with your elbow pointing forwards. This position will shorten your pectoralis muscles.

Using a slightly cupped hand, press your fingers into the muscle close to your shoulder. (Fig. 24a)

Slowly move your arm outwards so as to lengthen your pectoralis muscles while at the same time slowly dragging your fingertips through the muscle, towards your sternum. (Fig. 24b)

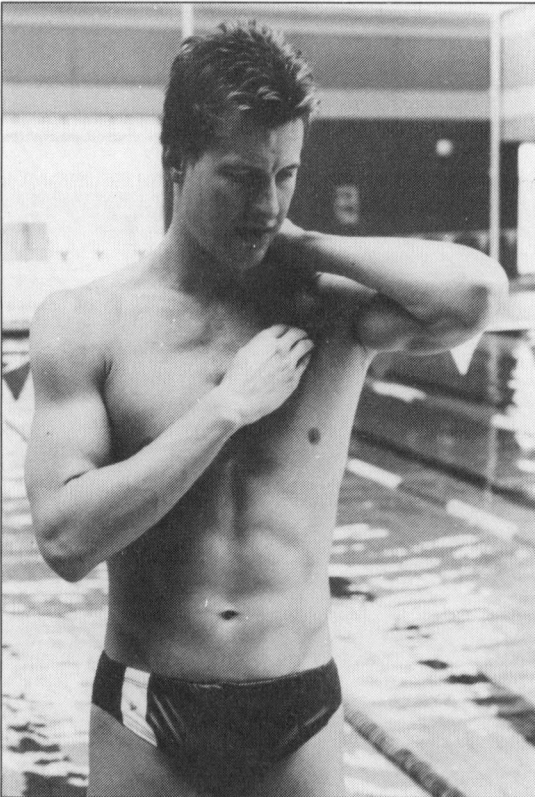

Fig. 24b

Fig. 24a

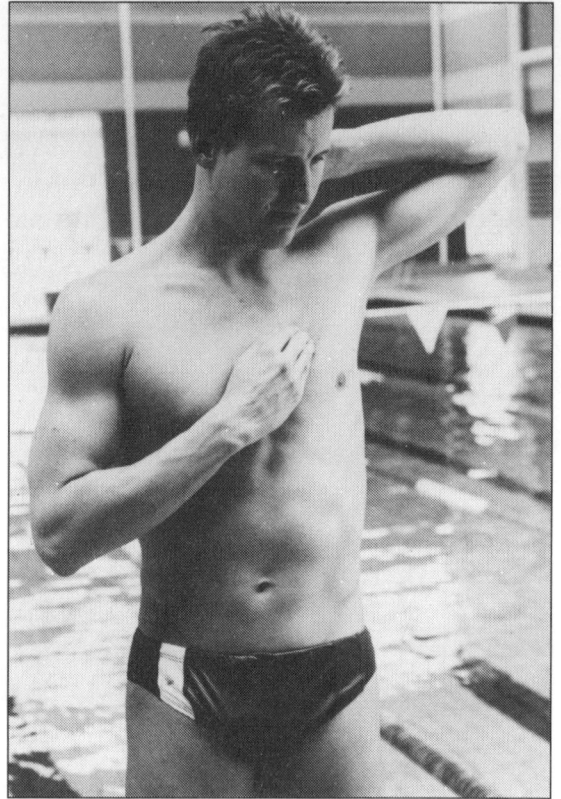

Biceps brachii

25.

Massage of both the long head and short head of the biceps begins with the arm to be massaged being flexed at the elbow.

Holding your arm, press your thumb into the muscle just above your elbow. Slowly push your thumb along the length of your biceps towards your shoulder. (Figs. 25a & b)

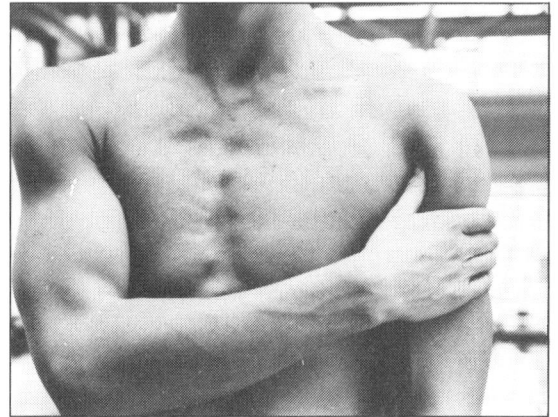

Fig. 25b

These long strokes will generally finish where the anterior deltoid muscle overlaps the upper part of your biceps.

Fig. 25a

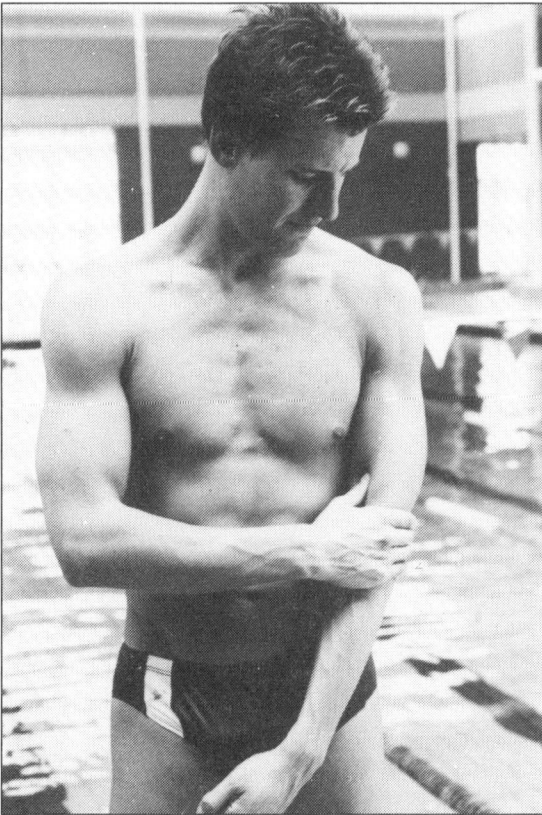

26.

To massage the musculotendinous junctions of the biceps, grip the inside of your arm so that your hand rests on the medial part of your biceps.

The musculotendinous junctions of the biceps lie just inferior to the anterior deltoid and will feel fibrous and most likely quite tender.

To massage this area transversely, press your thumb lightly at first into the musculotendinous junction and rock it back and forth. (Fig. 26)

Fig. 26

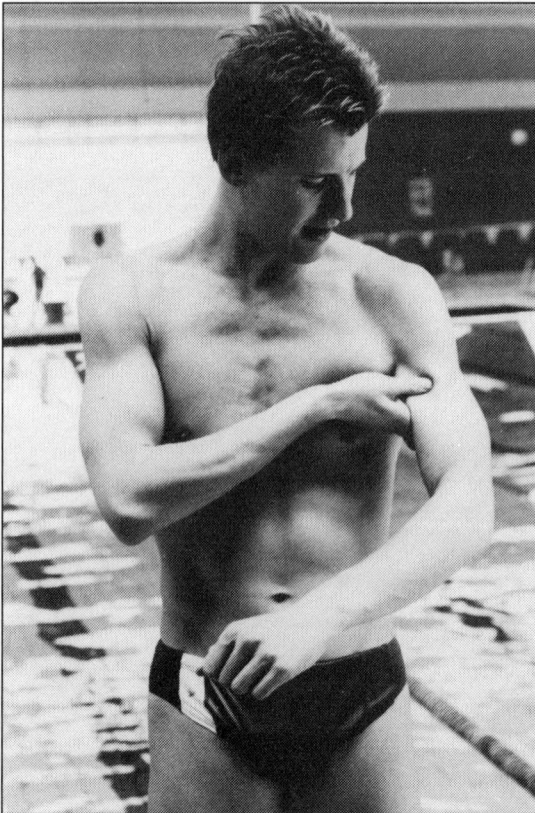

27.

Anterior shoulder pain is often caused by inflammation of the long head of the biceps tendon.

This tendon can be identified as a band of tightness running upwards along the front of the shoulder. It lies beneath the anterior deltoid and when inflamed will feel painful on palpation.

There are two simple techniques used for massaging the long head of the biceps tendon.

With your hand holding the outside of your shoulder, press the flattened pad of your thumb into the muscle on top of the tendon. Slowly push your thumb upwards, running along the length of the tendon. Each stroke will finish at the top of the shoulder. (Fig. 27)

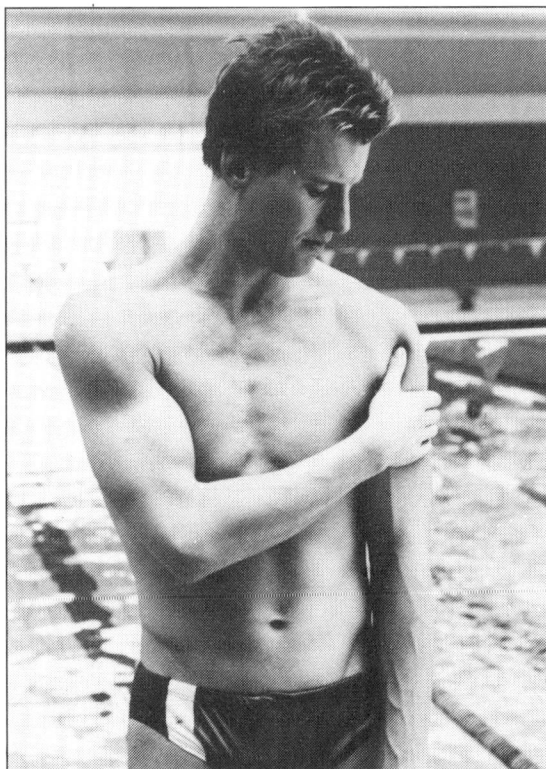

Fig. 27

The second method is to press the pads of your middle three fingers into the muscle over the part of the tendon you wish to massage. Rock your fingers backwards and forwards so as to perform transverse frictions over the tendon. The best results are achieved by using both these techniques.

Triceps

28.

Placing your forearm in front of your body, stand with the arm to be massaged bent at an angle of 60–90°.

Hold your arm so that the tips of your fingers are pressed firmly into your triceps. Slowly pull your fingers down towards your elbow while at the same time slowly straightening your arm. Repeat until your triceps have been thoroughly massaged. (Figs. 28a, b, c, d)

You may notice that the area just above your elbow is a little sensitive. This is where the three heads of the triceps converge to join a common tendon.

When stroking this tendon you may feel more discomfort than when you are massaging the muscle tissue of the triceps. It may therefore be necessary to reduce the pressure of the strokes slightly as they approach the elbow.

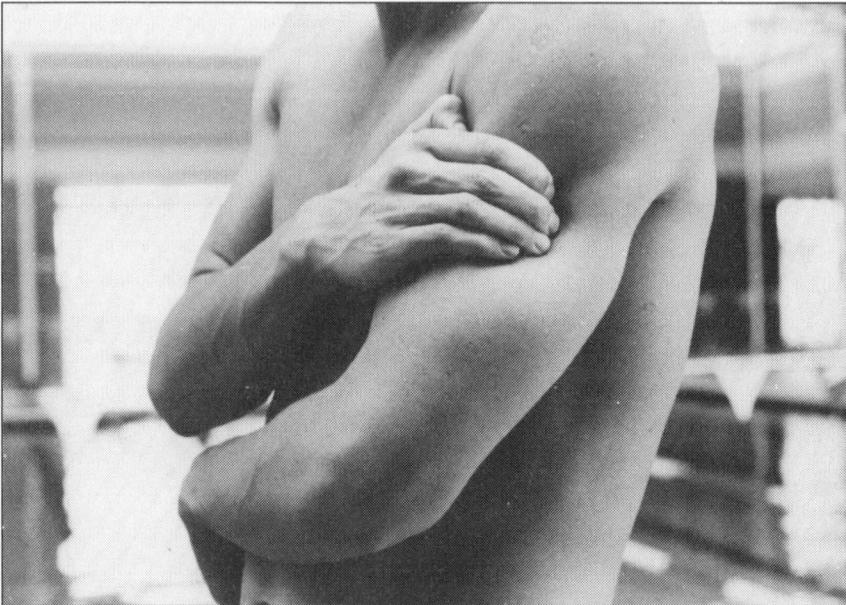

Fig. 28a

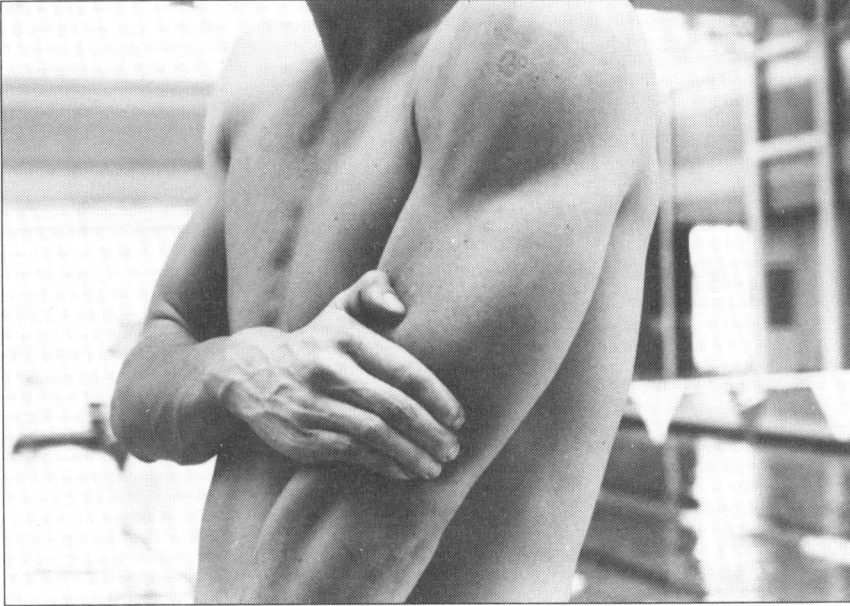

Fig. 28b

**Below left:
Fig. 28c**

Below: Fig. 28d

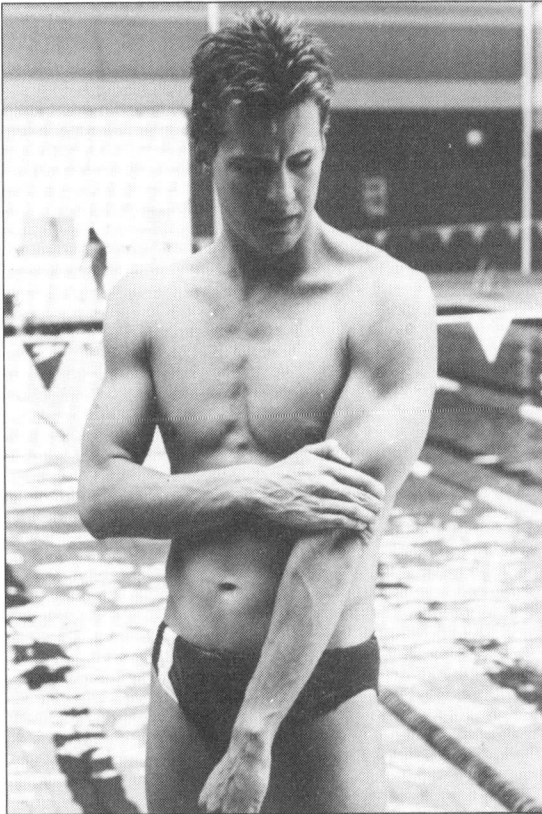

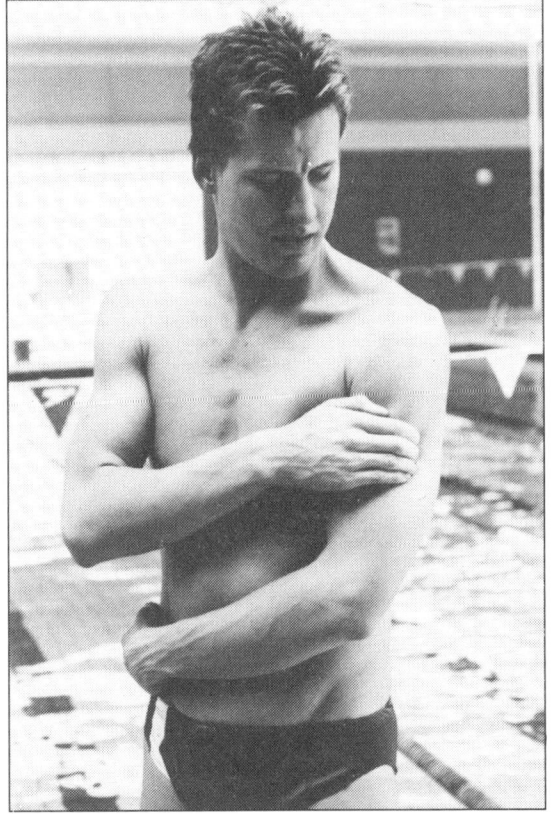

Forearms

29.

Press your thumb into the tissues just above your wrist. Gripping your forearm with your whole hand, push your thumb towards your elbow. (Fig. 29a)

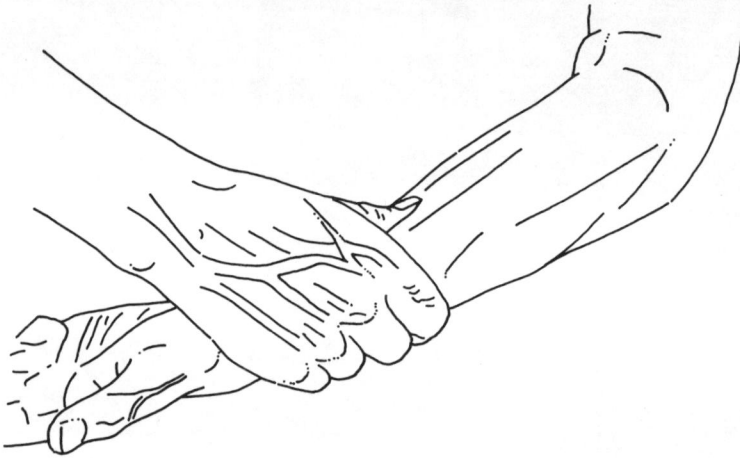

Fig. 29a

All of the muscles of your forearm can be thoroughly massaged by simply holding your forearm in various degrees of pronation (palm down) and supination (palm facing upwards) as the strokes are performed. (Fig. 29b)

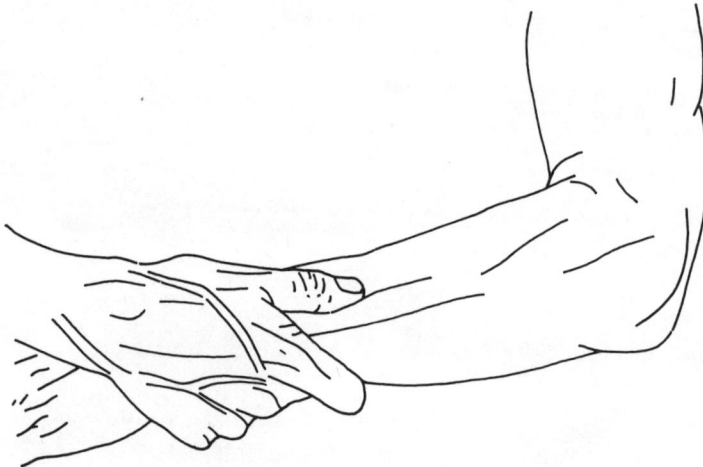

Fig. 29b

30.

Most of the muscles on the anterior surface of the forearm are responsible for flexing the wrist and fingers. You may find areas of tightness which have not responded satisfactorily to the longitudinal massage strokes. For these stubborn areas a very strong pressure technique can be used.

Begin with your hand open and wrist straight. Press your thumb firmly into an area of tightness and maintain the pressure as you slowly clench your fist. (Fig. 30a) Then slowly flex your wrist while continuing to maintain your thumb pressure and hold this position for several seconds. (Fig. 30b) Complete the procedure by slowly straightening your wrist, opening your hand and removing the thumb pressure. Repeat two or three times over each area.

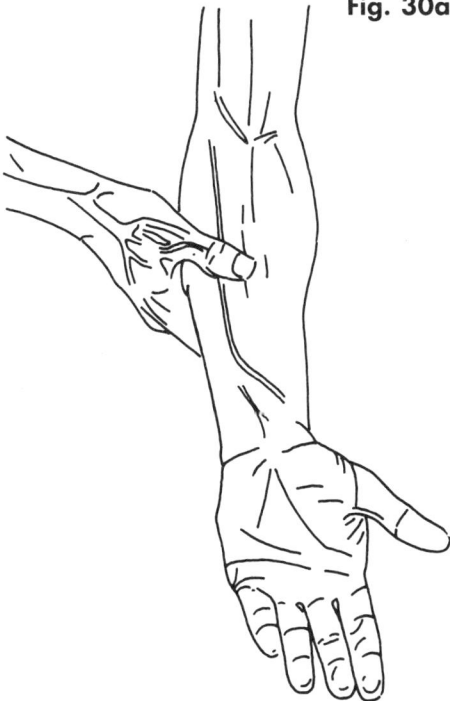

Fig. 30a

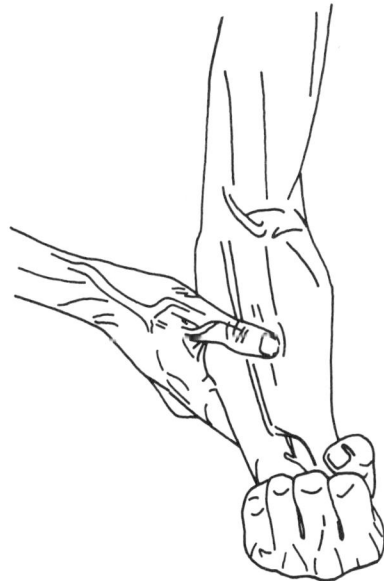

Fig. 30b

The muscles of the dorsal surface of the forearm can be massaged deeply using the same technique, but incorporating wrist extension.

Feet

31.

Sore and tired feet can be soothed by rolling a tennis
ball backwards and forwards under the arch of your foot.
This is best done while sitting down. Pressure is simply
determined by how hard you press on the ball. (Fig. 31)

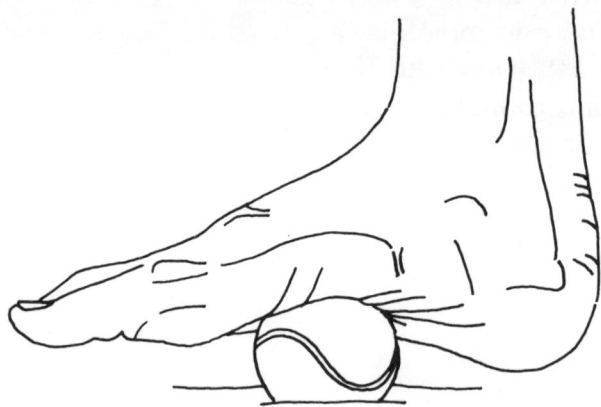

Fig. 31

32.

A simple acupressure technique can be applied to the
sole of your foot by holding it in both hands and using the
pads of your thumbs to apply point-pressure. Hold each
point for three to four seconds and work in lines from the
ball of your foot towards your heel. (Fig. 32)

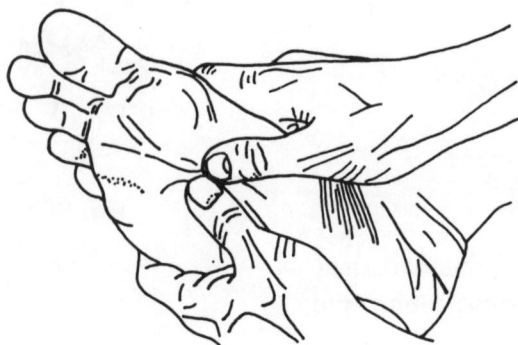

Fig. 32

33.

Friction can be used to relieve tightness by pressing your thumbs into the muscle and pushing them backwards and forwards, moving a few centimetres in each direction. Use a light pressure to begin with as feet can be very sensitive. (Fig. 33a)

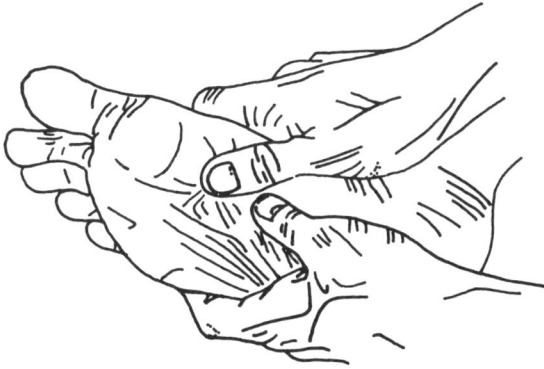

Fig. 33

Similar frictions can be performed across the top of your feet. (Fig. 33b)

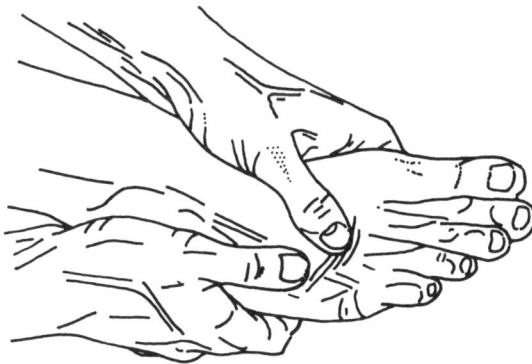

Fig. 33b

Hands

34.

Holding one hand with fingers slightly spread, gently squeeze areas of tightness and discomfort with the thumb and forefinger of the other. (Fig. 34)

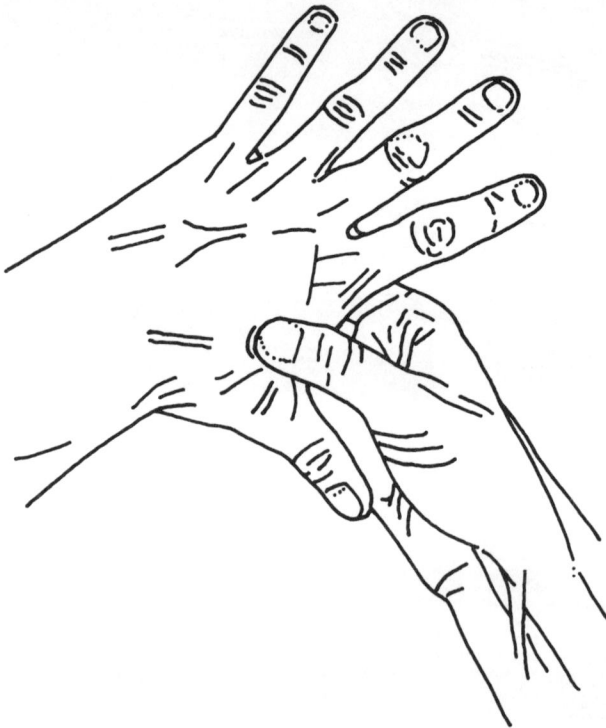

Fig. 34

By exerting pressure for several seconds, releasing the pressure, re-positioning your thumb and forefinger and then repeating the procedure, the entire area of your hands can be thoroughly massaged.

Certain areas will be particularly sensitive and warrant a more gentle pressure.

A backwards and forwards motion of your thumb and forefinger can also be used to massage particular areas.

35.

Interlock your fingers, holding the hand to be massaged so that its palm is facing upwards. With the thumb of your top hand, apply a direct downward pressure into points on your hand, holding each pressure-point, for three to four seconds. (Fig. 35)

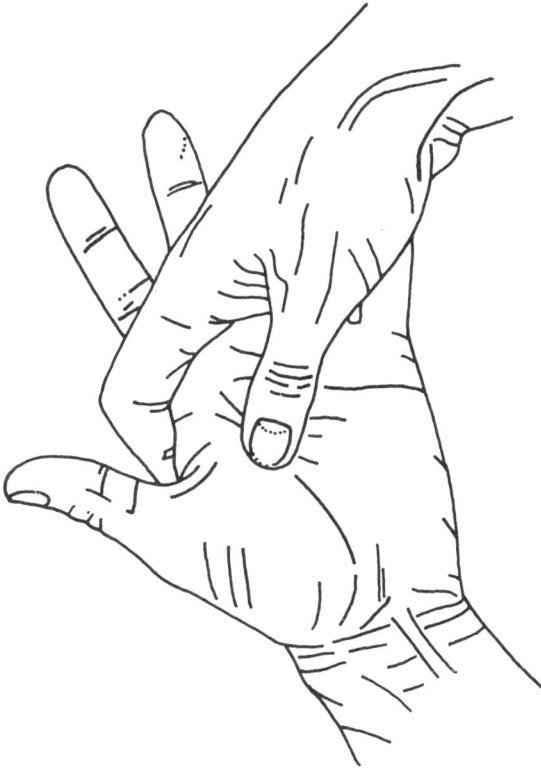

Fig. 35

You can also massage the surface of your hand by pressing your thumb into the other hand and slowly pushing it forwards, repeating the stroke many times.

The same technique can be used to massage the back of the hands by interlocking your fingers with the hand to be massaged facing palm down.

STRETCHING

Stretching

Very few athletes, even at a top level, use stretching to its fullest advantage, yet its benefits are too significant to be ignored. This chapter, therefore, outlines a comprehensive stretching program which can be adapted to the demands of particular sports.

Stretching plays an important role in the prevention of injury. Loss of muscle elasticity as a result of reflex-shortening and scarring can render you unduly susceptible to injury. Stretching before training or competition in order to lengthen muscles and get them functioning at an optimal level is essential to minimising soft-tissue trauma caused by vigorous exercise.

Stretching after exercise, when the soft tissues are still warm, will help reduce fatigue, facilitate quicker recovery and improve flexibility.

If the muscles cool after exercise without being stretched, they shorten and become tight. Stretching during the period of cooling-down will leave the muscles in an elongated state and the warm-up period in the next session will be noticeably more comfortable and productive.

To work out which stretching methods suit you best, it will help to have some understanding of the myotatic reflexes. These are two types — the stretch reflex and the inverse stretch reflex, which involve two types of receptors, muscle spindles and the golgi tendon organs.

The stretch reflex operates in the initial phase of stretching. When a muscle is stretched the body's immediate reaction is to prevent overstretching, by the muscle involuntarily contracting. This helps explain the sensation of tension experienced when adopting an initial stretch position.

Muscle spindles, which are sensitive to a change in length as well as the rate of change in length of the muscle fibre, transmit impulses more frequently to the spinal cord with stretching. This in turn increases the frequency of motor nerve impulses returning to the muscle, causing it to contract and resist elongation.

The inverse stretch reflex prevents the muscle tissue from being overstressed by too much tension from active contraction or excessive stretching.

Once the body has reached a point of tension, if the stretch position is maintained a 'draining' sensation may be experienced whereby the tension within the muscle slowly dissipates and the range of movement can be increased.

This results from the activation of the golgi tendon organs, which are located in the musculotendinous junctions of muscles. These have an inhibitory effect on the motor impulses returning to the muscle, thus allowing it to relax.

Stretching should be related to a particular sport and the requirements of each individual should determine the methods used. Stretching muscles which have not been suitably warmed up can cause injury.

All stretching procedures should therefore be preceded by a mild warm-up aimed at increasing muscle blood-flow, the lubrication of joints and generally raising body temperature. This should include low-level activity relevant to the sport being played, but also incorporating dynamic ranges of movement.

The five basic methods of stretching comprise static stretching, stretch- relaxation, passive stretching, proprioreceptive neuromuscular facilitation (PNF) and ballistic stretching.

Static Stretching

This is perhaps the most common form of stretching. Slowly stretch a muscle or muscle group as far as you comfortably can. Hold for 10–30 seconds, then release and repeat the procedure.

Greatly increased flexibility can be achieved by using static stretching at the completion of training or competition, before the muscles have cooled.

This technique is popular because it takes relatively little time. However, you should first warm up and take care not to cause an adverse muscular reaction by stretching too rapidly.

Static stretching should be regarded only as part of general warm up procedures.

Stretch-Relaxation

This is the safest method of stretching. You slowly go through a range of motion until you reach a point where you feel mild tension. This tension is likely to be a combination of the activation of the stretch reflex and pre-existing muscle tightness. At this point you maintain the stretch position until you have a sensation of tightness being drained from the muscles. The stretch position will then feel more comfortable to hold and the range of motion can be slowly increased until mild tension is again experienced. Repeat the process until you achieve maximum range of motion.

While stretch-relaxation may be a little more time-consuming, it is considered more effective than static stretching for improving flexibility.

Passive Stretching

This technique is used by extremely flexible athletes like gymnasts and requires the assistance of a partner to apply additional pressure to an area being stretched so as to be able to move through extreme ranges of motion.

Passive stretching requires not only the full co-operation of one's partner but considerable concentration, as there is a very real possibility of stretching the soft tissues beyond their limits and causing injury.

Proprioreceptive Neuromuscular Facilitation (PNF)

This is another form of partner-assisted stretching which has clear advantages but also certain disadvantages.

Greatly improved flexibility can be achieved using PNF stretching.

During the initial phase of the PNF technique, slow passive stretching is carried out with the assistance of a partner. Once a point of mild muscle tension is reached, indicating the activation of the stretch reflex, a subsequent agonist and/or antagonist muscle contraction of approximately three seconds is used to produce stimulation of the golgi tendon organs. This of course inhibits the spindle cell impulses returning to the muscle being stretched. The range of motion can be further increased with a second passive stretch manoeuvre.

The main disadvantage of PNF stretching lies in the fact that it requires the assistance of a partner.

Ballistic Stretching

Ballistic stretching may not be as effective as other techniques for improving flexibility, but it does generate heat within the muscles and lubricates joints, thereby preparing them for the dynamic actions essential in many sports where the athlete moves quickly in and out of near end-of-range stretch positions.

Ballistic stretching is characterised by bouncing or jerking actions (eg alternate toe touches), and should only be used as part of the final preparation to training or competition, once a suitable warm-up and stretching routine has been completed.

Incorrectly performed stretching can damage soft tissues and many athletes have inadvertently turned an injury-prevention practice into the cause of an injury by overstretching.

Indications of overstretching are muscle tension which becomes greater the longer the stretch is held, and vibrating or quivering of the part of the body being stretched. Should these reactions be experienced, the stretch should be slowly released and subsequent stretches approached more cautiously.

To sum up, there are a number of important points to remember when developing a stretching program:

Precede stretching with a relatively effortless warm-up of approximately five minutes.

Stretch before and after exercise.

Select stretching techniques and exercises that are most suited to your sport.

Go into each stretch slowly and in a controlled manner and come out of it the same way.

During stretching, your breathing should be slow, deep and rhythmical.

Do not make unrealistic demands of yourself by trying to emulate other people who may be more flexible than you are.

It is desirable to do some stretching after self-massage. The muscles will be warm as a result of increased muscle blood-flow and will benefit even more from a short period of stretching. I recommend stretch-relaxation combined with static stretching at this time.

Spend a few minutes using the stretch-relaxation technique until you reach a maximum stretch position that feels comfortable. Complete the procedure by holding this position with a static stretch of approximately thirty seconds.

Stretching

1. Neck and upper fibres of trapezius

Taking hold of your elbow or forearm behind your back, gently pull your arm downwards so that your shoulder is depressed. Slowly tilt your head to the opposite side until you feel mild tension down the side of your neck and across the top of your shoulder. (Fig. 36)

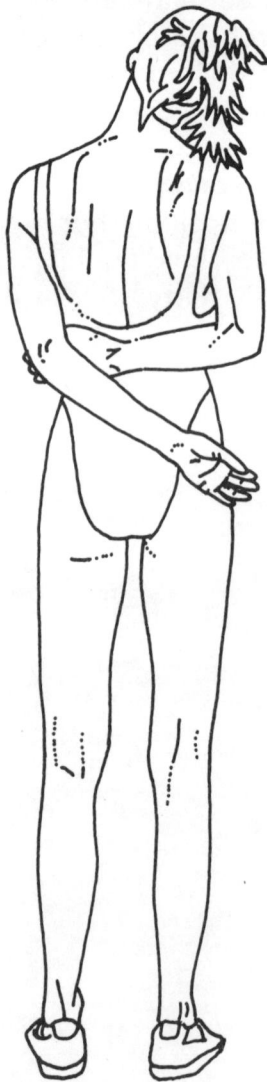

Fig. 36

2. Triceps

With your arm raised, take hold of your elbow and gently pull it across behind your head until you feel mild tension along the back of your arm. (Fig. 37)

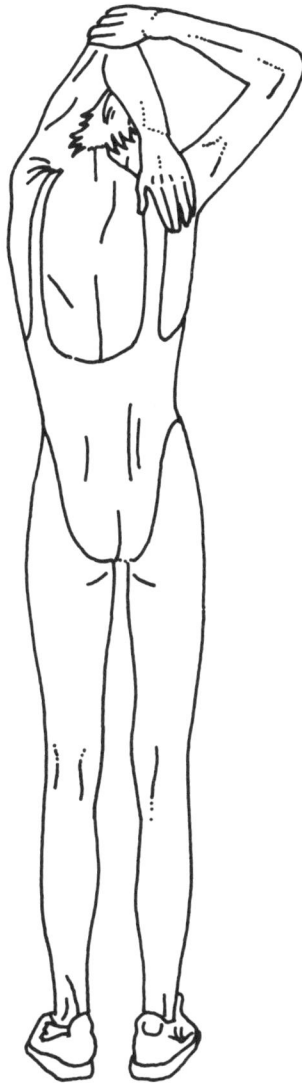

Fig. 37

3. Rhomboids and lower fibres of trapezius

Sit on the floor with your knees bent so that your feet are resting flat on the ground. Pass your arms behind your knees and take hold of your elbows. Lowering your head towards your knees, gently draw your shoulder blades backwards, using your arms for resistance.

You will feel mild tension between your shoulder blades. (Fig. 38)

Fig. 38

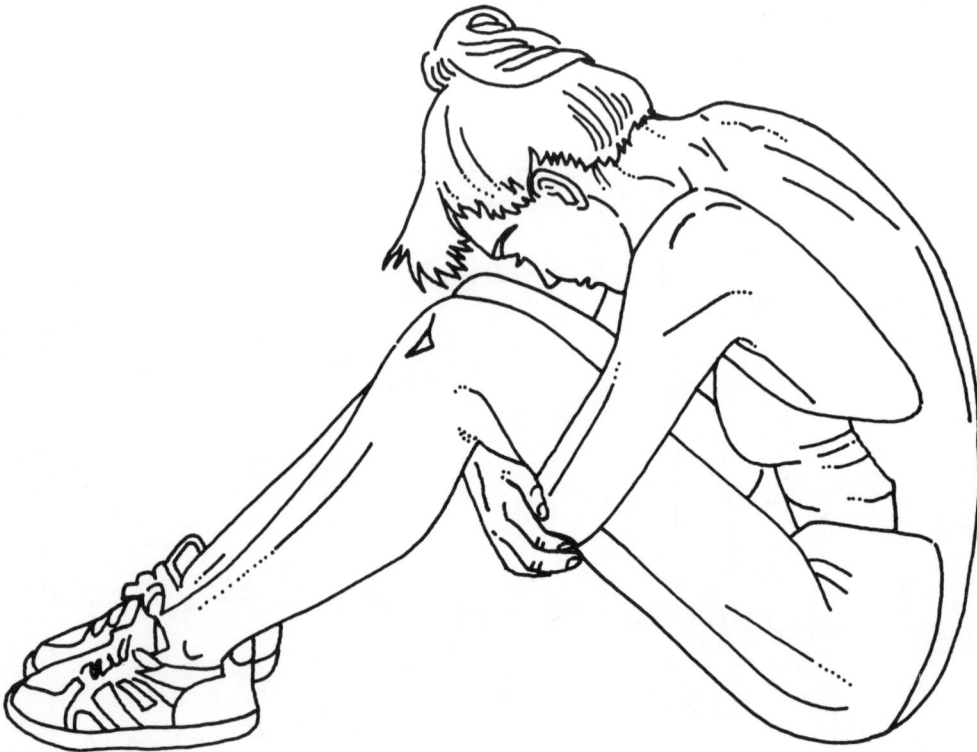

4. Pectoralis muscles and biceps brachii

Standing side-on to a wall, flatten your arm against it horizontally behind you. Slowly move your body position away from the wall until you feel tension across your chest and along the front of your arm. (Fig. 39)

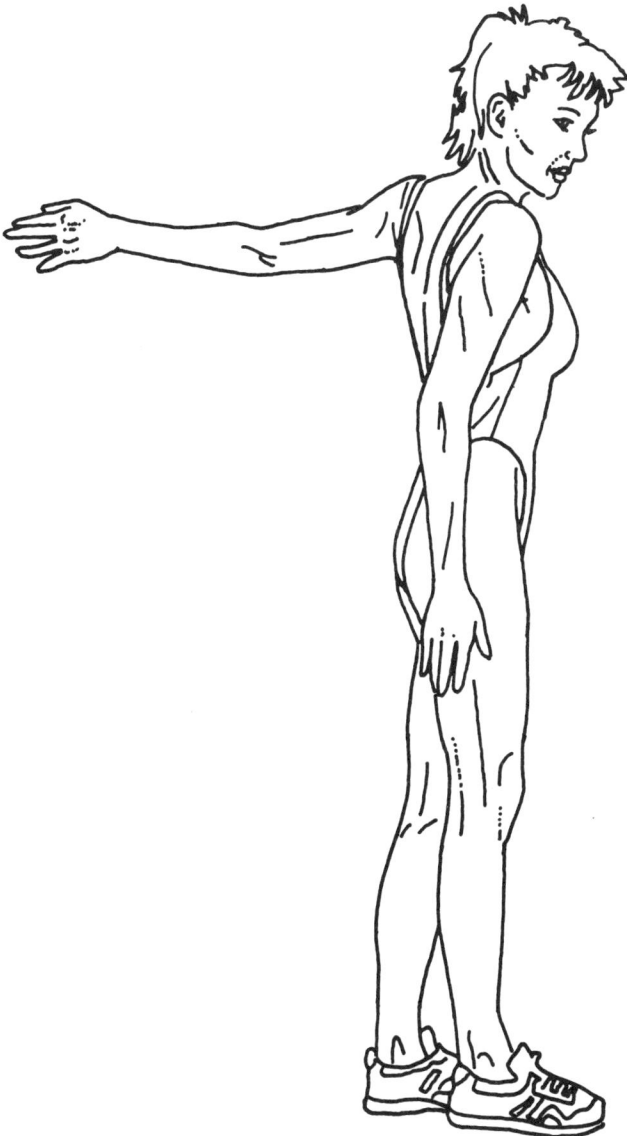

Fig. 39

5. Biceps

Hold your hands with the palms facing upwards and your elbows locked behind your back. Keeping your body upright, slowly raise your arms until you feel tension along the front of your shoulders and down your arms. (Fig. 40)

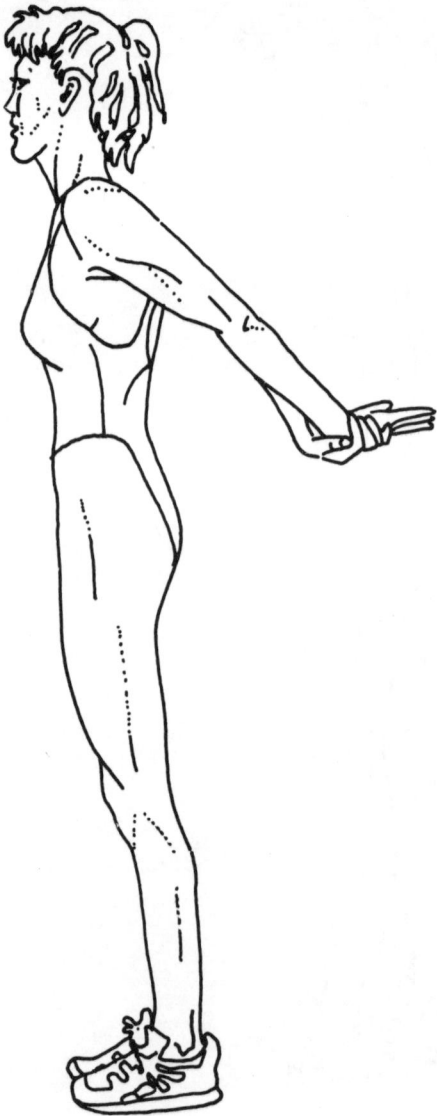

Fig. 40

6. Infraspinatus

Holding one arm at the elbow, gently pull it across your chest until you feel tension behind your shoulder and across your shoulder blades. (Fig. 41)

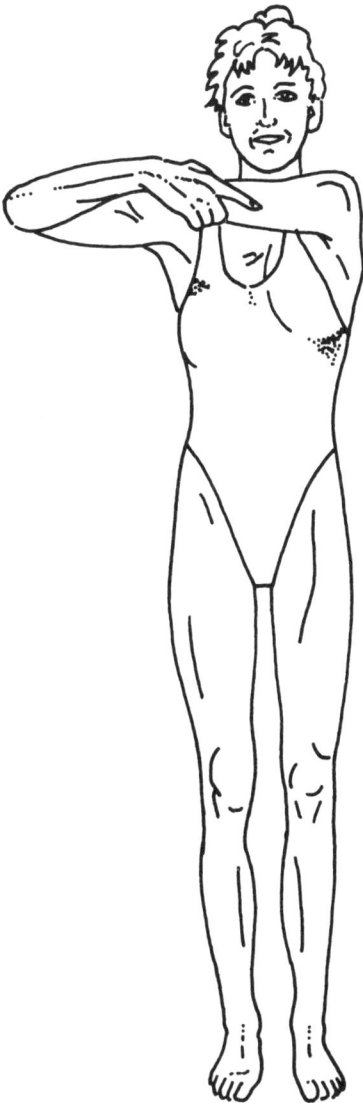

Fig. 41

7. Latissimus dorsi

Bending at the waist, reach forward with your arms fully extended to take hold of a structure at approximately waist height. Allow the weight of your upper body to drop downwards so that you feel stretch behind your shoulders and along your sides. To increase stretch, roll the upper part of your body first to one side and then to the other. (Fig. 42)

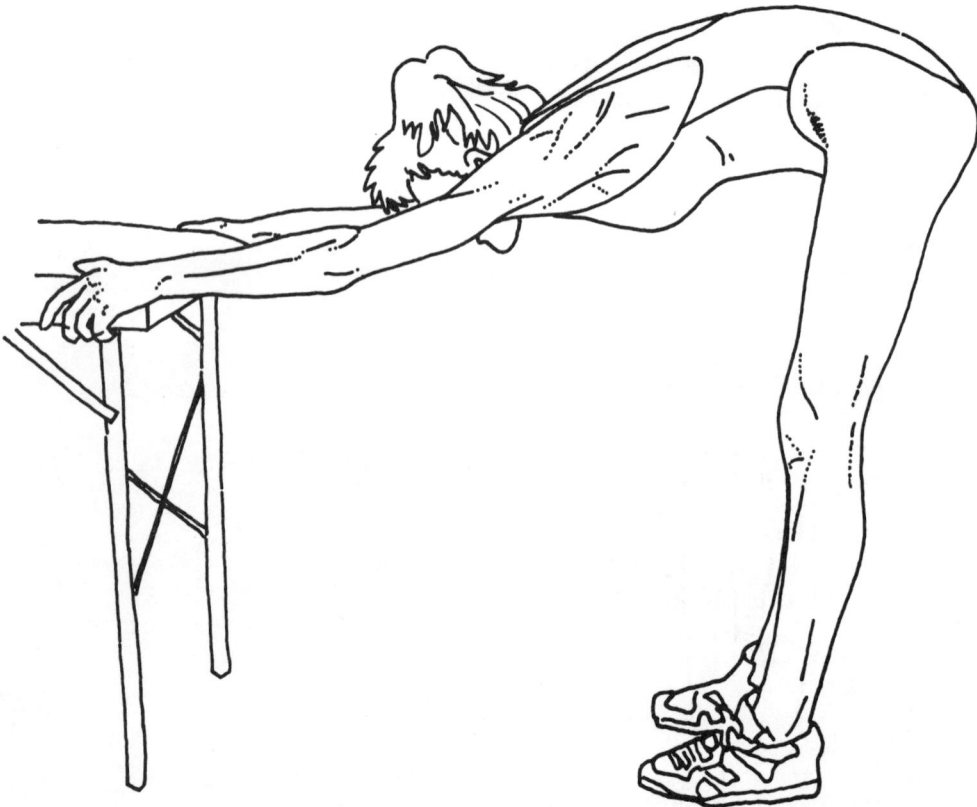

Fig. 42

8. Lower back and gluteal region

Lie on your back with your knees bent so that your feet are resting flat on the ground. Slowly drop your legs towards the ground, alternating from one side to the other. (Figs. 43a & b)

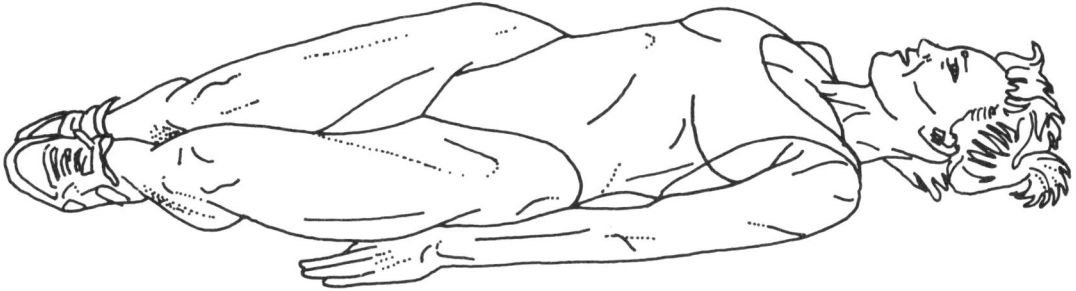

Fig. 43a

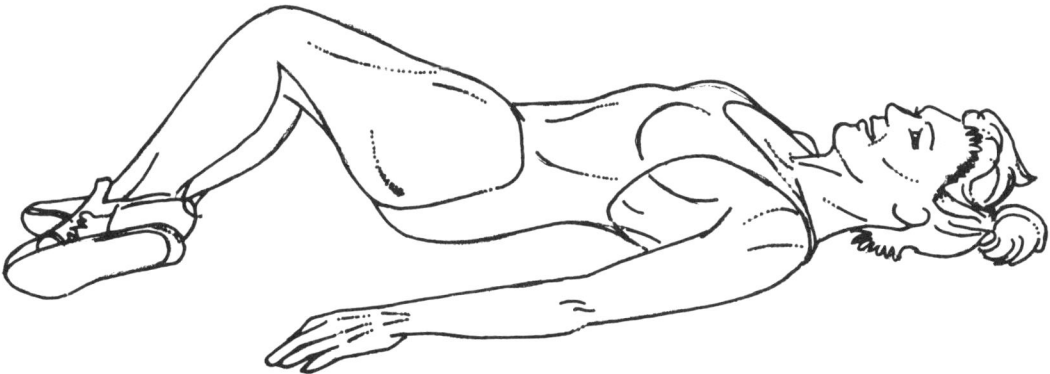

Fig. 43b

9.

Sitting on the ground, place your left foot on the outside of your right knee. Use your right elbow to push against the outside of your left knee while at the same time rotating your upper body to the left.

Use the opposite procedure to stretch your other side. (Fig. 44)

Fig.44

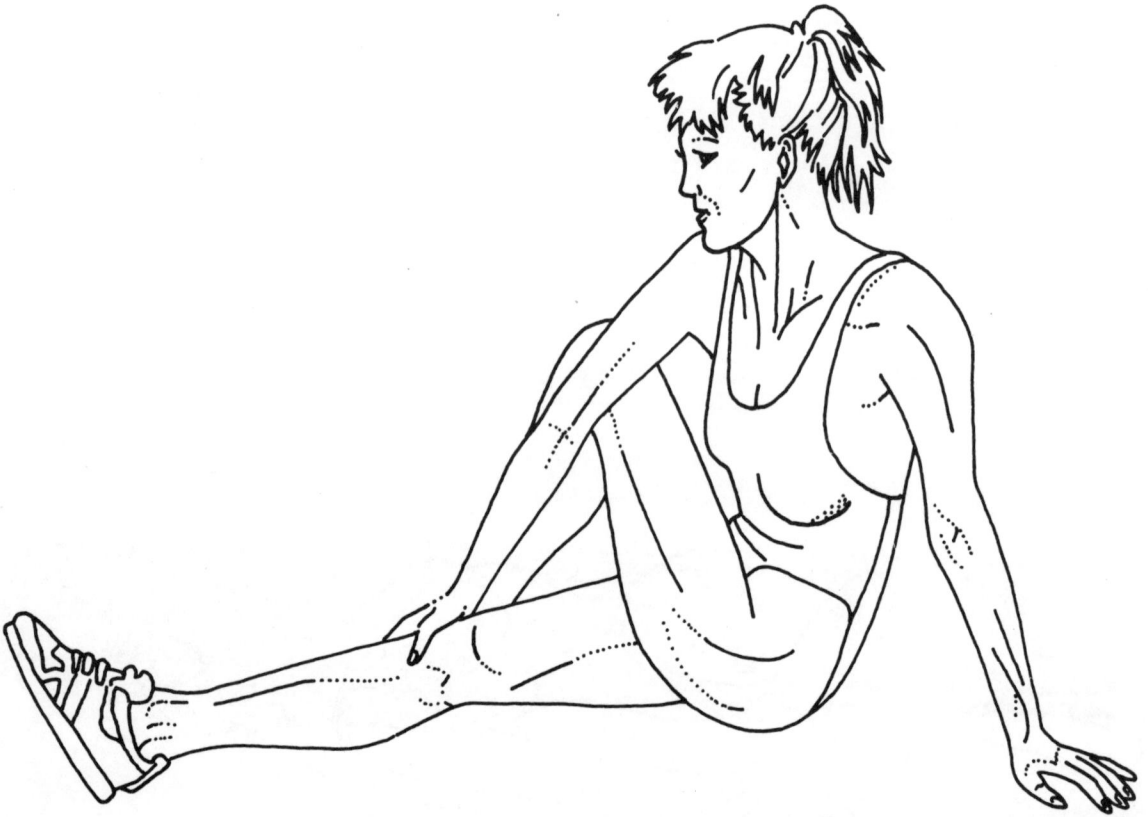

10.

Sitting on the ground, take hold of your left knee with your left hand and your left ankle with your right hand. Slowly draw your left foot towards the midline of your body until you feel mild tension in your buttocks.

Use the same procedure to stretch the other side. (Fig. 45)

Fig. 45

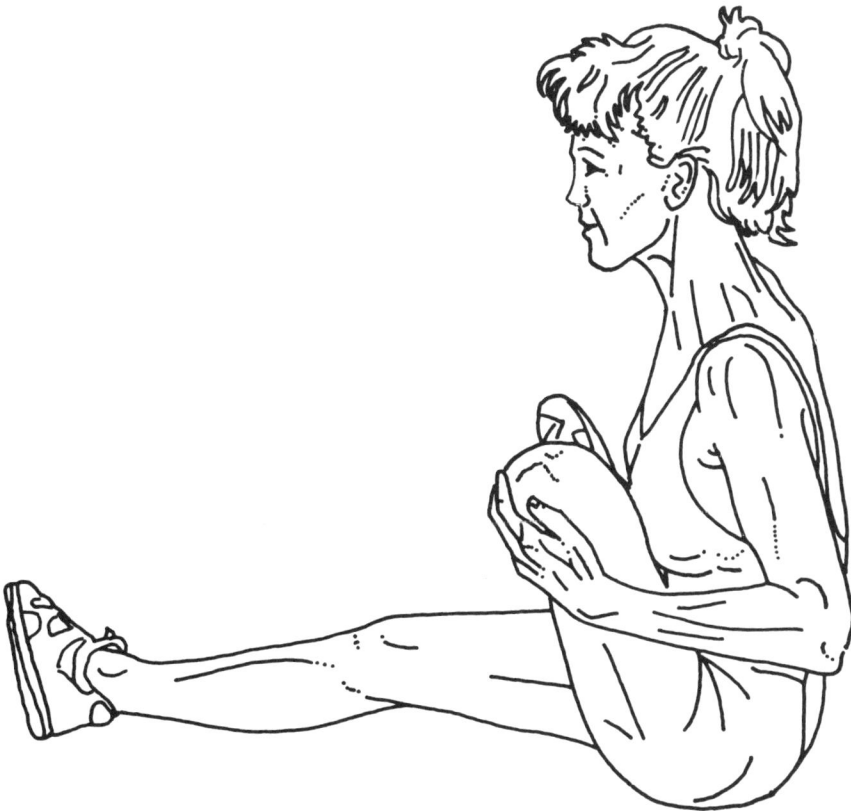

11.

Position yourself on your hands and knees. To stretch the right side of your buttocks, place your right hand slightly forward of your left hand. Keeping your left knee locked, place your left foot across and behind your right foot. Slowly rotate your right hip towards the floor until you feel mild tension in your right buttock. (Fig. 46)

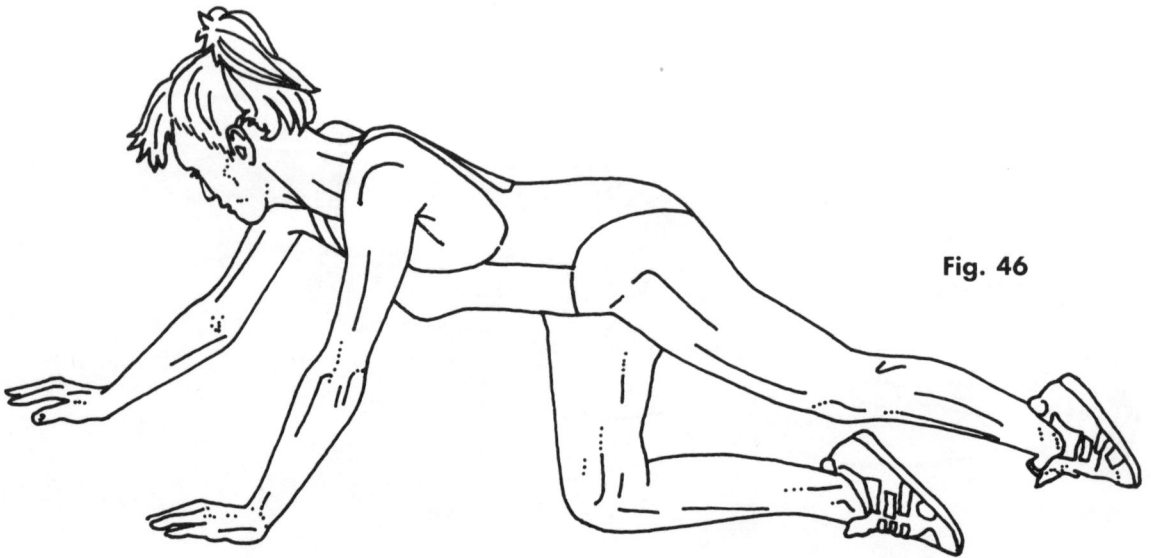

Fig. 46

12. Quadriceps

Standing upright, take your foot in one or both hands
and slowly draw it up towards your buttocks. Do not allow
your body to lean forward as this will make the stretch less
effective. (Fig. 47)

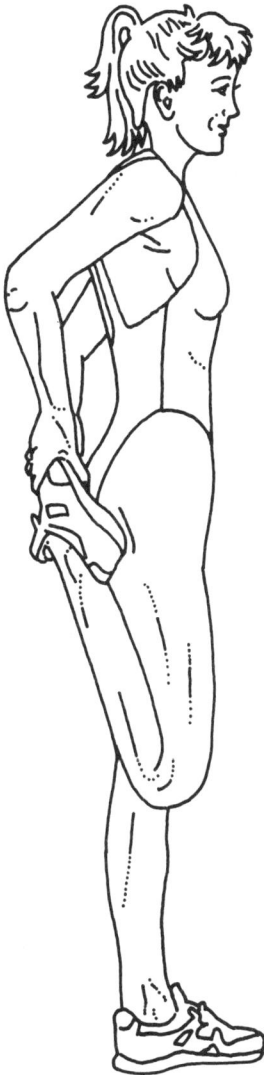

Fig. 47

13. Hamstrings

With your leg extended at an angle of approximately 90°, lean your body forward. Bend from your hips rather than curling your back. (Fig. 48)

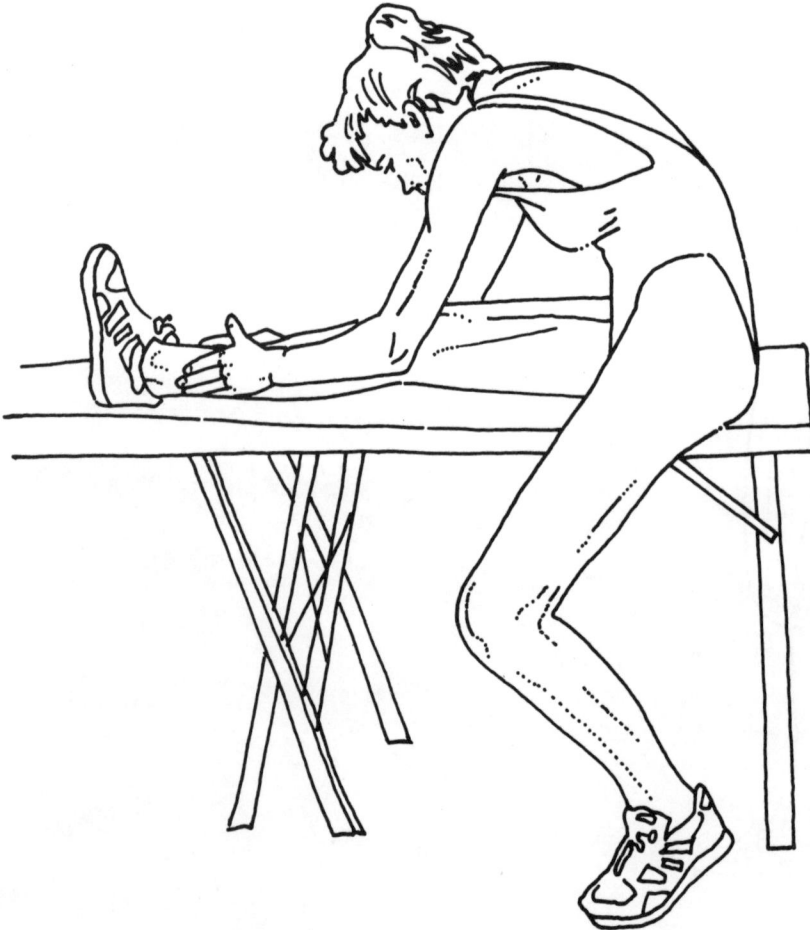

Fig. 48

14. Adductors

Sit on the floor with your feet drawn towards the midline of your body, with the soles held together. Use your elbows to apply downward pressure over your knees until you feel mild tension through your groin and adductors. (Fig. 49)

Fig. 49

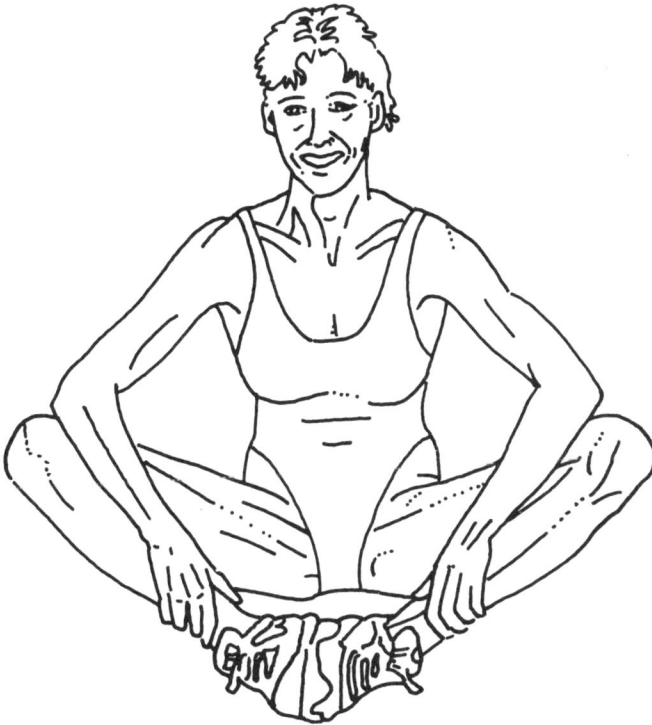

15. Calves

a. Push against a wall, keeping your back foot flat and knee straight. (Fig. 50a)

b. To stretch deeper muscles, slowly bend the knee of your back leg while continuing to keep your foot flat on the ground. (Fig. 50b)

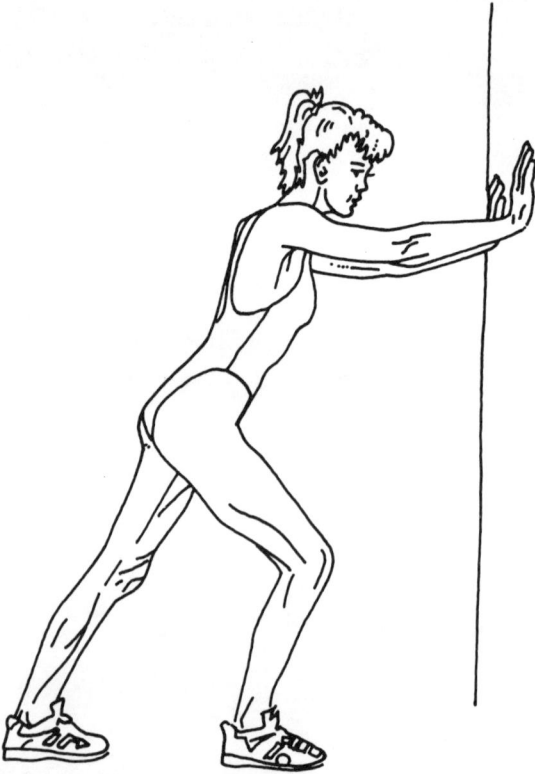

Fig. 50a

Fig. 50b

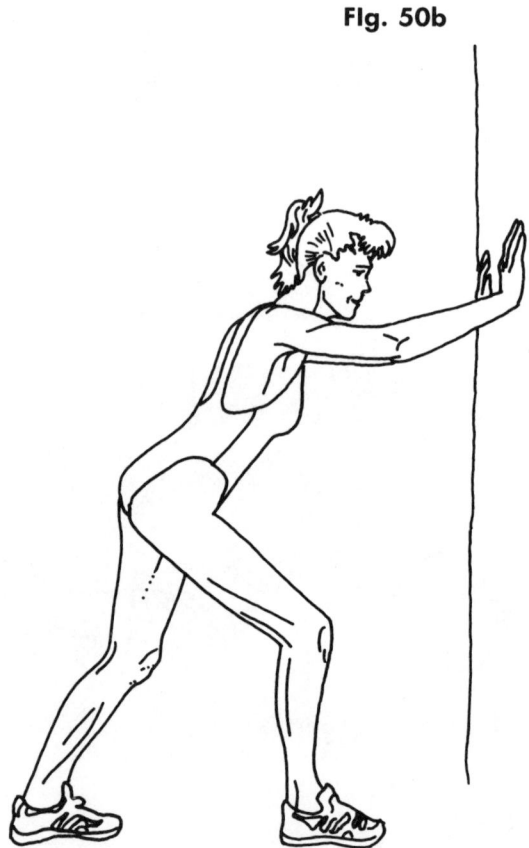

c. To stretch calves and Achilles tendons further, squat
over your left leg, keeping your toes in line with your right
knee. Keeping your left foot flat on the ground, slowly
lean your body over your left leg to the point at which the
heel of your left foot begins to lift from the ground.
(Fig. 50c)

Reverse position to stretch the calf and Achilles tendon
of your right leg.

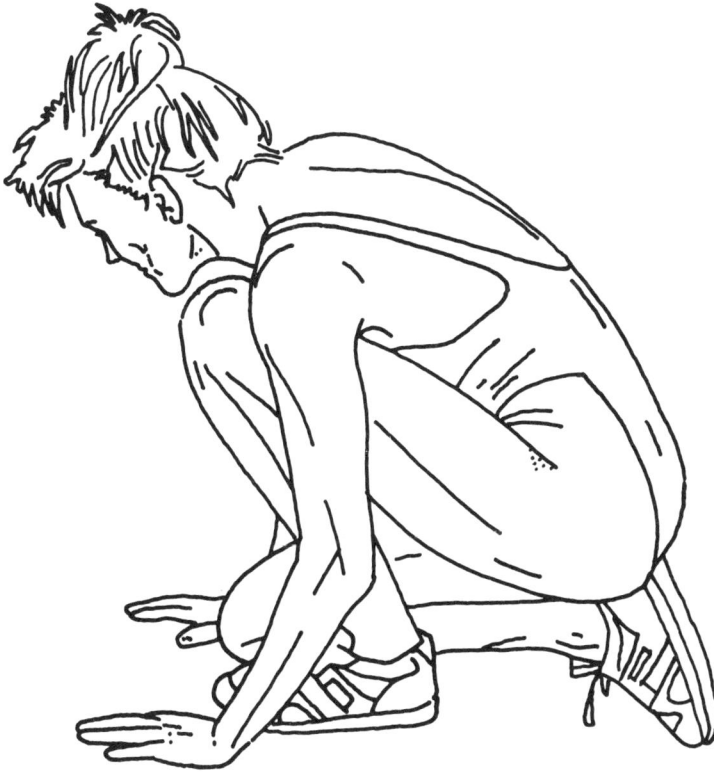

Fig. 50c

Ice and Heat in Injury Treatment

Many people are unsure of the physiological effects of hot and cold treatment for injuries, and how and when they should be applied.

With any soft-tissue injury, you should seek proper advice as soon as possible. But, there are certain steps you should take straightaway to minimise tissue damage and the time lost before you're able to resume normal training and activity.

The greatest contraindication of massage comes when it's applied to recently traumatised tissues. If it's applied too soon to the injured spot, its mechanical action and the fact that it increases local blood supply will cause greater bleeding from capillaries into the tissue spaces, the removal of more intracellular substances from damaged cells and a larger inflammatory response.

Heat also increases muscle blood-flow, and should not be applied during the first 48–72 hours following injury. Instead, the affected tissues should be immediately cooled by the use of ice.

Cooling the tissues causes vasoconstriction, resulting in a reduction of blood-flow. Vasoconstriction is touched off by a shrinking of the blood passageway within the capillaries and by the action of the precapillary sphincter, situated at the point where capillaries branch off from the metarterioles, controlling the flow of blood to a particular area of tissue.

Cooling the tissues also lowers their metabolism, reduces the formation and leakage of intracellular substances from damaged cells, and generally restrains inflammation.

Ice is beneficial not only straight after injury but also during recovery by easing residual pain.

Muscles respond to pain by involuntarily contracting to immobilise and protect the injured area in a sustained spasm which can cause further soft-tissue damage by compressing the associated blood vessels and inhibiting the supply of vital oxygen and nutrients to the tissues.

Muscle spasm can also prevent the injured part returning to full mobility.

Ice applied to an area of muscle spasm may decrease pain by reducing nerve conduction in some of the smaller pain fibres and suppress the reflexes causing spasm, thereby allowing the muscles to relax.

The relief of pain by the application of ice will enable you to start sooner on a carefully structured exercise program necessary for full recovery. Although ice decreases circulation and slows down the metabolic process, these negative effects are more than compensated for during the rehabilitation phase by the beneficial effects of exercise. However, once pain has eased sufficiently for exercise to be resumed, the benefits of continuing to use ice are questionable.

The duration of its use depends to some extent upon the depth of the injury. The deeper the area the longer it takes for effective cooling to occur. Opinions vary on how long each application should last, but the usual period is about twenty minutes. During immediate post-injury treatment, applications may be frequent and longer.

Compression, elevation and rest are also necessary at this time. A close but not too tight elastic wrap should be worn for at least 24 hours and the injured part kept above the level of the heart.

According to a theory known as the 'Hunting Response', the body reacts by reflex to sustained applications of cold, during which periodic vasodilations (expansions of the blood passageway resulting in increased blood-flow) occur to prevent the tissues from being damaged by excessive cooling. This hypothesis has yet to be fully proved, but although blood-flow levels may fluctuate, it seems fairly certain that ice makes the capillaries less permeable, thus minimising the risk of further tissue damage from serous fluids (oedema).

Although massage and heat should not be employed in the initial treatment of soft-tissue injuries, they are valuable later in speeding up the healing process by increasing muscle blood-flow, which intensifies the interchange of nutrients and wastes. The application of heat, like ice, also eases pain by making the pain receptors less conductive and thus reducing muscle spasm.

The value of heat linaments is questioned by some therapists, who believe that while they may affect superficial tissues, their heat properties do not reach deep muscle-tissue but merely stimulate blood-flow and are dispelled from the body through the skin and by the lungs. It may be the massage that is used to rub these linaments into the skin which is most therapeutic.

The most effective form of specific heat treatment is thought to be the application of various physiotherapy electrical modalities and hot packs over the injured spot.

To summarise:

- R.I.C.E. — Rest, Ice, Compression and Elevation — should be applied during the first 48–72 hours following injury.

- The use of ice will facilitate an early resumption of therapeutic exercise by checking inflammation.

- The application of ice to areas of muscle spasm and pain can prevent secondary soft-tissue damage.

- Heat should not be applied during the first 48–72 hours following injury.

- Heat is useful for treating pain and muscle spasm during the phase of injury rehabilitation.

APPENDICES

APPENDIX 1: THE HUMAN BODY

I. The Muscular System

The muscular system, like all the systems of the human body, is extremely complex.

Muscles are controlled by the nervous system and are divided into three groups according to the type of nerve fibres they contain.

1 *Skeletal* or *voluntary* muscles — attached to bones and controlled by the central nervous system.

2 *Visceral* or *involuntary* muscles — located in the internal body structures and controlled by the involuntary or autonomic 'self-governing' nervous system.

3 *Cardiac* muscle — controlled by the autonomic nervous system and an independent 'pacemaker' mechanism, situated in the walls of the heart.

As far as the effects of massage on the body is concerned, the most important are the skeletal or voluntary muscles.

Skeletal muscles generally arise or insert themselves in bones. The point of attachment which does not move when the muscle contracts is known as the muscle origin, while the point which moves is known as the insertion. The point at which the muscle meets the tendon fibres (the musculotendinous junction) is frequently susceptible to injury.

Muscles vary in shape according to the arrangement of fibres on the muscle tendons. Nearly all the voluntary muscles are found in pairs and are named according to any one of six basic characteristics — their location, direction in which they lie, function, shape, numerical division or point of attachment.

Muscles are composed of a multitude of cylindrical parallel fibres, varying in length from 1 mm to 30 cm. Each fibre is made up of hundreds to thousands of tightly packed myofibrils consisting of protein molecules. The myofibrils are in turn composed of two kinds of myofilaments — thick ones called *myosin* and thin ones

Sports Massage and stretching

called *actin*. According to the 'sliding filament' theory, it is the friction of these myofilaments which is responsible for muscle contraction.

Once they cease contact, the muscle is able to relax to its original length.

Accompanying each muscle and muscle group are a number of connective tissue structures. These include the *endomysium* which surrounds each muscle fibre, while each bundle of muscle fibres is surrounded by the *perimysium*. The entire muscle is encapsulated within the *epimysium* and many muscle groups, particularly those of the lower limbs, are surrounded by a tough fibrous tissue called the *fascia*. Part of the muscle mass is thus made up of connective tissue.

It is possible that much of the tightness within a muscle comes from this extensive framework of connective tissue.

There are two types of muscle fibres, commonly known as 'slow twitch' and 'fast twitch'. 'Slow twitch' or red fibres tend to manifest themselves more in endurance athletes as they function aerobically, due to the fact that they are high in myoglobin which combines with oxygen from the bloodstream and transports it into the cells. They also have a high capillary density, and large quantities of fat, enzymes and mitochondria. The last produces adenosintriphosphate (ATP), which is a primary source of energy.

'Fast twitch' fibres, on the other hand, are white. They function anaerobically, as they are low in myoglobin, fat, enzymes and also mitochondria, which means they produce less ATP although at a much quicker rate. As well, they have a lower capillary density. Both fibre types are found in a single muscle, but the proportion of 'fast' and 'slow' will vary from person to person.

It is useful to understand how muscles function. An *agonist* is a muscle which contracts concentrically — i.e. the muscle shortens with contraction to produce movement. An *antagonist* muscle produces an opposite type of movement. For example, the biceps brachii (agonist) is responsible for bending the elbow, while the tricep (antagonist) straightens the elbow.

A *prime mover* is a muscle that plays the main role in producing a movement and can initiate that movement on its own. An *assistant mover* only helps with a movement once it has been initiated by a prime mover.

A *stabiliser* is a muscle which contracts isometrically (i.e. develop tension without shortening) to provide a firm, stable base on which another muscle can act. Finally, a *synergist* is a muscle which modifies an action initiated by another. For example, the hamstrings may act synergistically to slow the leg down towards the end of the movement after a ball has been kicked.

Muscles often become tight after vigorous exercise because of scarring and reflex-shortening. One of the great advantages of massage is its effectiveness in returning tight and shortened muscles to their optimal resting length. It also makes them more extensible, improves blood-flow and reduces muscle tightness.

What can massage achieve in terms of flexibility that a good stretching program cannot?

Tightness is not so often experienced equally throughout the full mass of muscle but in specific areas like points within the muscle belly or perhaps at a musculotendinous junction. Stretching is generally intended to elongate a complete muscle so it is therefore difficult to direct a stretch manoeuvre to a localised area.

Perhaps specific tightness within a muscle can be traced to the connective tissue structures. In this case massage can be applied more directly to the affected area and combined with appropriate stretching techniques to achieve optimal muscle extensibility.

II. The Circulatory System

The circulatory system is made up of the heart, blood vessels and blood itself.

The heart is a hollow organ approximately the size of a fist, situated between the lungs and resting on top of the diaphragm. Two-thirds of it lies to the left of the sternum,

which shields it at the front, while at the back it is
protected by the vertebrae.

The heart is composed of four chambers, the left and
right *atria* and the left and right *ventricles*, which together
act as a pump in circulating blood throughout the body.

The left side of the heart moves oxygen-rich blood to the
organs and muscles. The right side moves deoxygenated
blood to the lungs, where it is replenished with oxygen.

Oxygenised blood is transported at high pressure away
from the heart by thick-walled vessels called *arteries*. The
one exception to this is the pulmonary artery, which carries
deoxygenated blood from the heart to the lungs.

Deoxygenated blood is transported at low pressure back
to the heart by thin-walled vessels called *veins*. The only
exceptions are the pulmonary veins, which carry blood
newly replenished with oxygen from the lungs back to the
heart. Veins have valves which govern the flow of blood
and prevent it from coursing backwards and accumulating.

Deoxygenated blood enters the right atrium and passes
into the right ventricle, from which it is pumped to the lungs
to be resupplied with oxygen. From here the oxygen-
enriched blood enters the left atrium, passes into the left
ventricle and is then pumped away to the body via the
aorta, which is the main trunk of the arterial system.

From the aorta other major arteries branch off to give
rise in turn to a myriad network of ever-diminishing
auxiliary vessels — first the *arterioles*, then the
metarterioles and finally the *capillaries*, which are
responsible for the transport of blood through the tissues.

Following the exchange of oxygen and nutrients, the
capillaries drain into small veins called *venules*. The
venules increase in size until the blood — now depleted of
oxygen and nutrients — reaches the veins, by which it is
then carried back to the heart.

The principal function of the blood, which is vital to all
the tissues of the body, is transportation. Oxygen and
nutrients are carried to the cells, and carbon dioxide and
waste matter away from them. These wastes are taken to
the kidneys, which are part of the urinary system and are

responsible for the excretion of harmful substances. Other functions of blood include the regulation of pH (the acid-base balance of body tissues), body temperature and the water-content of cells.

Two of the benefits of massage relevant to the circulatory system are its ability to assist venous blood-return and increase muscle blood-flow, both of which have significant effects upon the recovery and regeneration of muscle-tissue following exercise.

III. The Lymphatic System

The tissues of the body are bathed in interstitial fluid which acts as a medium for interchange of nourishment and waste products between the circulatory system and the body tissues.

Interstitial fluid leaks from the capillaries and is primarily plasma which is the substance making up 55–60 per cent of the blood.

Following the interchange of nutrients and waste, interstitial fluid drains into the vessels of the lymphatic system where it is referred to as lymph.

Lymph vessels begin as closed-end tubules situated in spaces between the cells, which unite to form larger channels. These channels form an extensive network throughout the body similar to the circulatory system. They resemble small veins, and like veins they have valves which control the flow of lymph.

The lymph vessels lead to a series of nodes or glands — situated chiefly in the neck, groin, thorax, armpits and abdomen — which act as a filter for the lymph. These nodes contain lymphocytes which produce antibodies and are responsible for the destruction of bacteria and other foreign bodies which may have invaded the tissues and been drained into the lymphatic vessels.

Lymph may pass through several groups of nodes before it is actually returned to the bloodstream. Ultimately the lymphatic vessels drain into the junction of the left and right subclavian veins beneath the collarbone and the left and right internal jugular veins which unite to form the innominate veins. These drain into the superior *vena cava*, which is the major vessel entering the right side of the heart. Blood passes to the right ventricle and is pumped to the lungs where it is reoxygenated, and so the cycle continues.

There is a constant circulation of lymph from the capillaries into the tissue spaces, back into the lymph vessels and returning to the blood.

Damage to muscle cells as a result of injury will result in intracellular fluid and some cellular components draining into the tissue spaces, while damage to capillaries will make them more permeable and result in bleeding into the tissue spaces. The consequent increase in interstitial fluid will cause the tissues to swell, creating the condition known as oedema. Normally, however, the lymphatic vessels will drain excess interstitial fluid and return it to the circulatory system.

Though there does not appear to be any scientific evidence that massage assists the functioning of the lymphatic system, it is generally felt that swelling within the soft tissues can be reduced through what is termed 'lymphyatic drainage'. The tissues are massaged in a direction consistent with that of the lymph vessels returning towards the heart, so that interstitial fluid is drained into them and localised swelling is reduced.

Regardless of the circumstances, a medical specialist should always be consulted whenever oedema occurs. There are many possible causes of this disorder, for some of which massage would possibly be an inadvisable treatment.

IV. The Nervous System

The nervous system consists of two main parts — the *central*, comprising the brain and spinal cord, which interprets information from external sources and co-ordinates the body's response; and the *peripheral*, which is found everywhere else in the body and connects receptors with the central system.

Efferent nerve cells carry information from the brain and spinal cord to all parts of the body. They divide into two groups — the *voluntary* (or somatic), which is responsible for controlling the muscles, and *involuntary* (or autonomic).

The involuntary or autonomic nervous system is further divided into the *sympathetic* and the *parasympathetic* systems, which interact to control automatic bodily functions. The peripheral nervous system is therefore endlessly gathering and transmitting data to the central system and causing the body to react to its signals.

Nerves are in fact single cells that are usually found in great numbers and arranged together so as to form a *nerve cord*. When we speak of nerves we usually really mean nerve cords. These cords conduct impulses which cause activity upon reaching their destination. If the destination is a muscle, for instance, the resultant activity may be contraction and, ultimately, movement.

Again, there is little research on massage relating to the nervous system, but it is generally considered that light to mild massage will stimulate the nerves, while heavy pressure will sedate them.

For this reason only light, brisk, strokes are used in administering massage immediately before vigorous exertion, to arouse the muscles to a state of readiness, whereas afterwards deeper and more rhythmical massage is applied in order to relax and calm them.

V. Muscles

Muscles of the chest

Pectoralis major — this thick, triangular muscle situated at the front of the chest arises from the sternum or breastbone and the anterior surface of the sternal half of the clavicle (collarbone). It inserts itself by way of a thick, flat tendon into the head of the humerus at the top of the arm. (Fig. a)

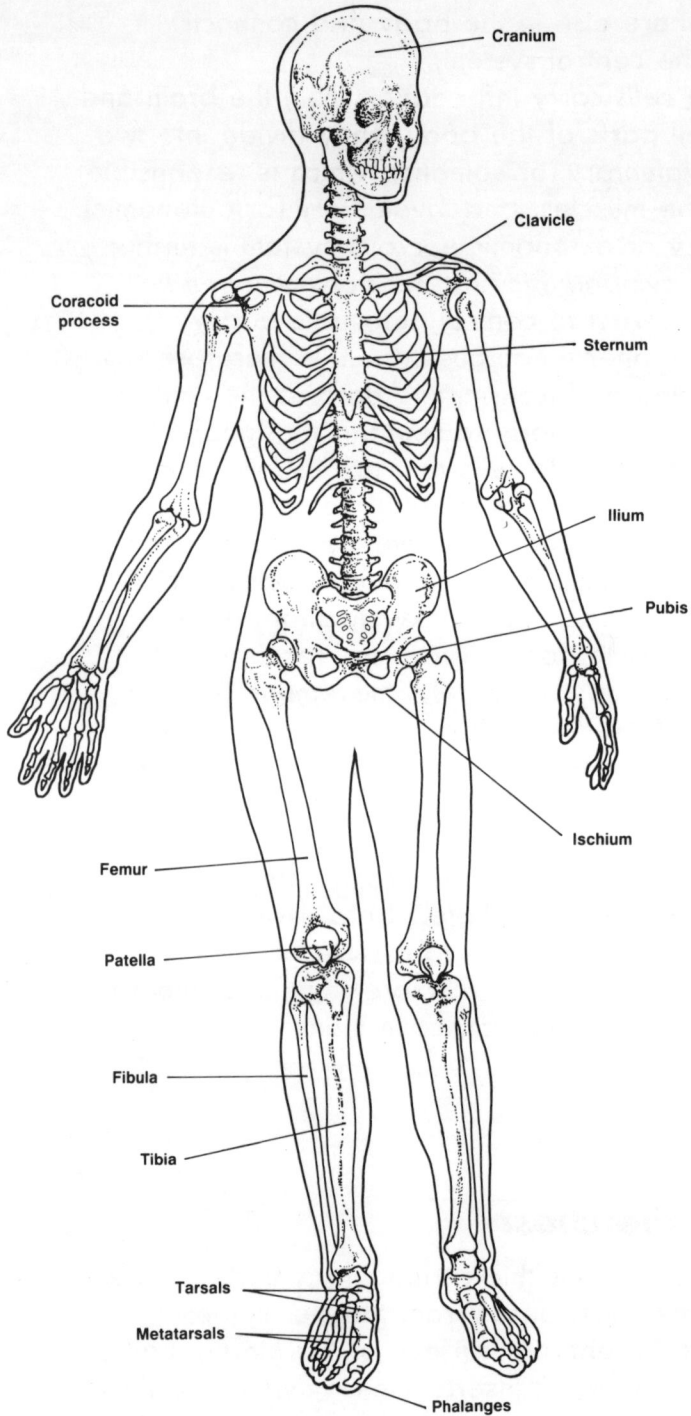

Front view of the human skeleton.

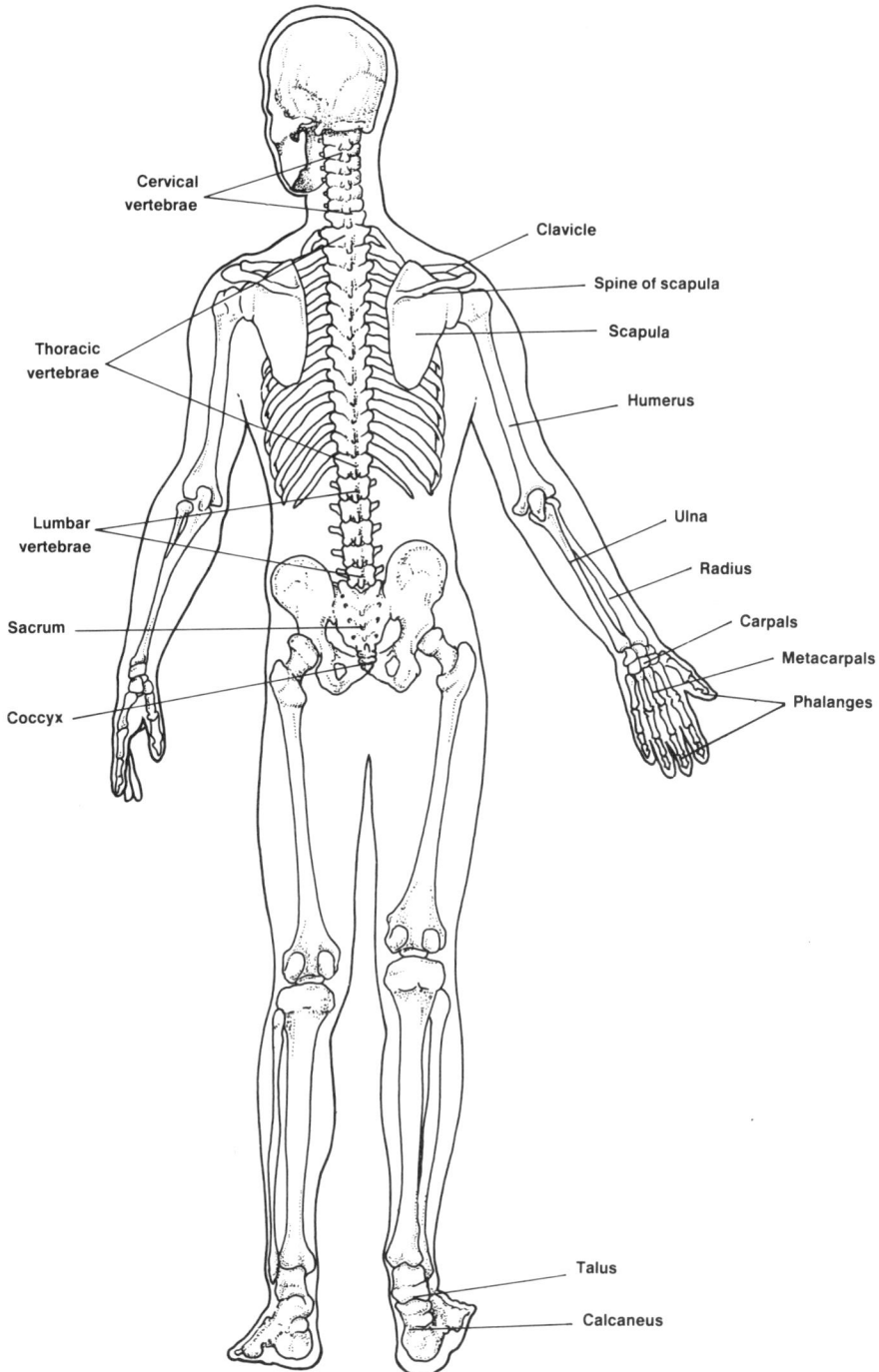

Cervical
vertebrae

Clavicle

Spine of scapula

Scapula

Thoracic
vertebrae

Humerus

Ulna

Lumbar
vertebrae

Radius

Sacrum

Carpals

Metacarpals

Phalanges

Coccyx

Talus

Calcaneus

Back view of the human skeleton.

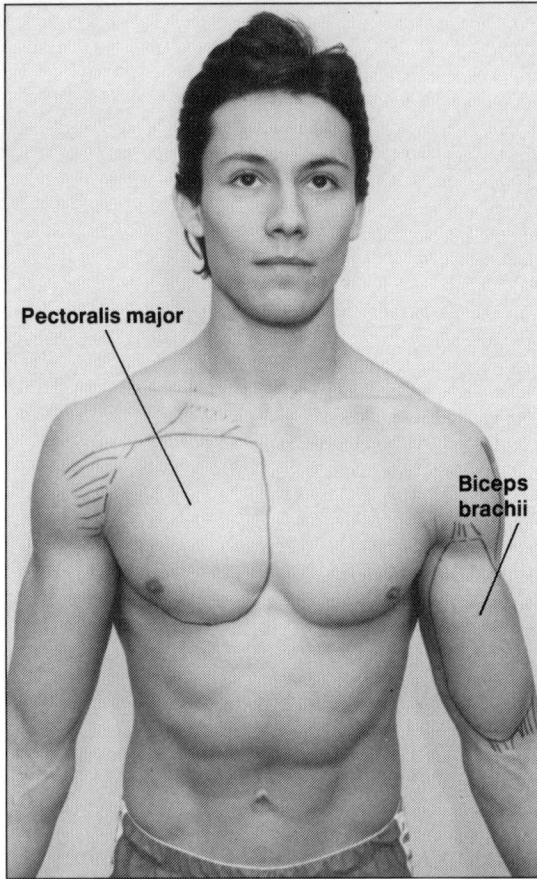

Fig. a

Pectoralis minor — a thin, triangular muscle situated deep to the pectoralis major. Much of it arises from the third, fourth and fifth ribs and inserts itself into the bony coracoid process of the scapula (shoulder-blade).

Muscles of the shoulders and upper back

Trapezius — a broad, flat, triangular muscle, placed immediately beneath the skin and fascia, and covering the upper and back part of the neck and shoulders.

Supraspinatus — lies beneath the upper fibres of the trapezius and occupies the space of the scapula above its spine. The fibres of the supraspinatus converge to attach to the top of the humerus. (Fig. b)

Infraspinatus — a thick triangular muscle which covers the posterior surface of the scapula below its spine. Part of the infraspinatus is covered by posterior deltoid and its fibres converge to insert themselves into the humerus.

Latissimus dorsi — a broad flat muscle which arises from the crest of the ilium near the pelvis, the vertebrae of the sacrum behind it, and the lower and middle back. The extensive network of fibres of the latissimus dorsi taper and converge, crossing the lower point of the scapula and attach to the humerus.

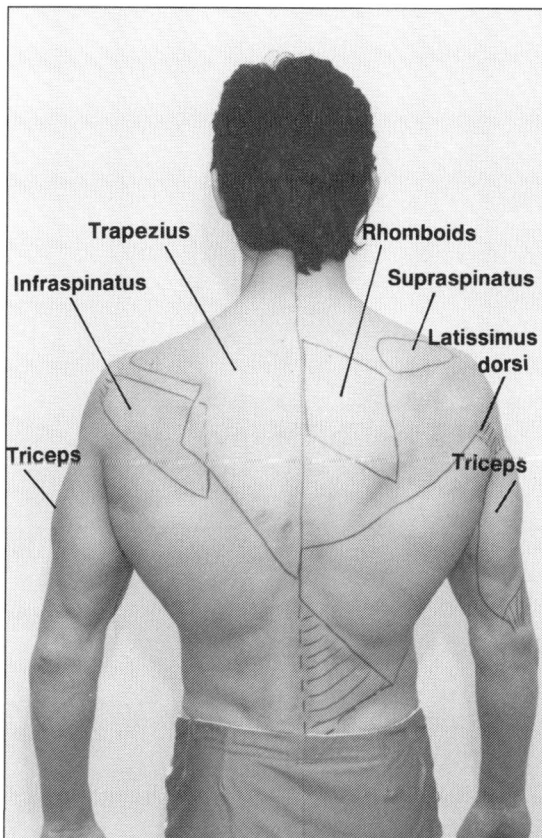

Fig. b

Rhomboids — this pair of muscles lies beneath the lower fibres of the trapezius and arise from the lowest cervical vertebrae near the neck and the first five thoracic vertebrae below them. They lie on a downwards angle to attach to the medial border of the scapula.

Muscles of the arms

Biceps brachii — a long muscle made up of two portions, at the front of the arm. It arises from two different features towards the top of the scapula and attaches at the top of the radius, just below the elbow.

Triceps — made up of three portions and occupies the length of the back of the humerus. It arises from a point on the scapula and most of the back of the humerus and attaches just below the elbow onto the ulna bone of the forearm.

Muscles of the forearms

For ease of explanation most muscles of the forearm can be divided into two groups. *Flexors*, situated on the anterior surface of the forearm, are responsible for flexing the wrist and fingers. They are the gripping muscles. At the posterior of the forearm are the *extensors*, responsible for extending the wrist and fingers and so releasing grip.

Muscles of the thigh

The *quadriceps* include four individual muscles (Fig. c):

Vastus medialis — arises from a prominent ridge along the middle third of the femur or thighbone and inserts itself into the inner border of the patella (kneecap) and the quadriceps tendon.

Rectus Femoris — situated in the middle of the front of

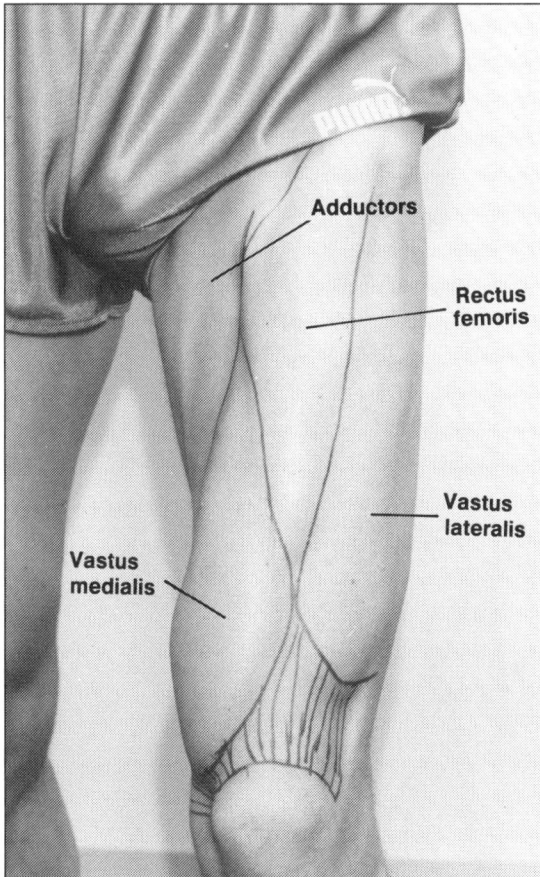

Fig. c

the thigh and attached to the patella. It arises from two tendons, one connected to the front of the ilium and the other into the rim of the bony prominence on which the head of the femur sits.

Vastus Lateralis — the largest of the quadricep muscles, situated on the outside of the thigh. It arises from points at the top of the femur and inserts itself by way of a flat tendon into the outside of the patella.

Vastus Intermedius — cannot be seen as it lies deep to the other quadriceps muscles. It arises from the upper two-thirds of the front of the femur and forms a deep part of the tendon that attaches to the top of the patella.

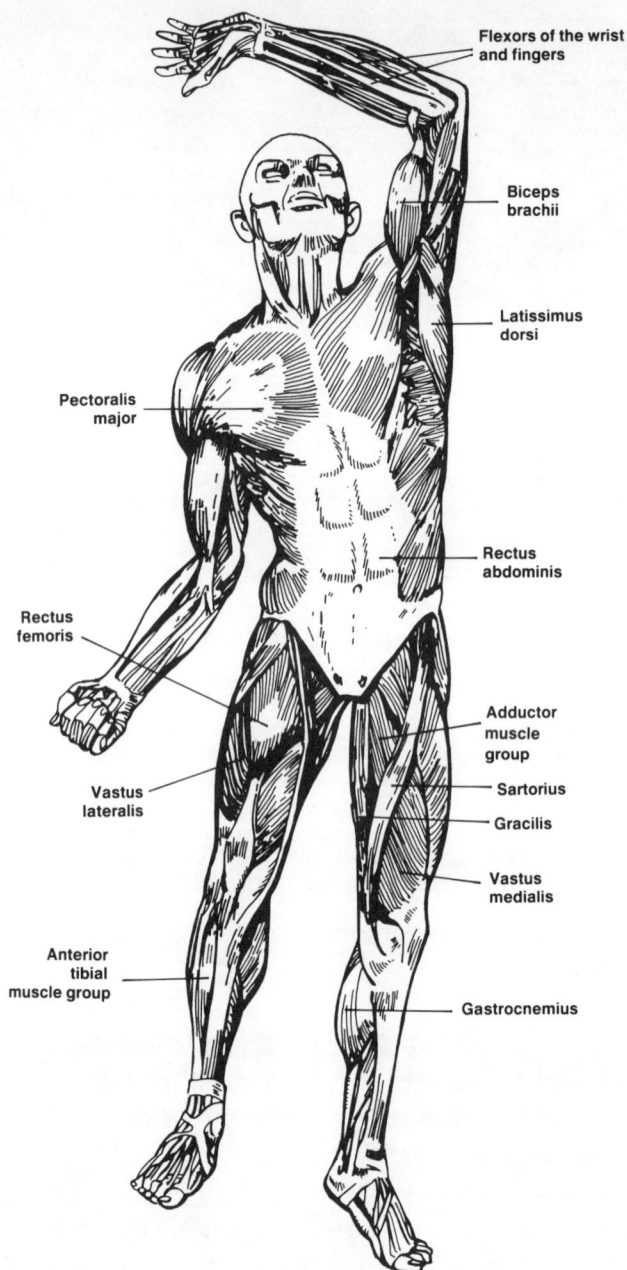

Flexors of the wrist and fingers

Biceps brachii

Latissimus dorsi

Pectoralis major

Rectus abdominis

Rectus femoris

Adductor muscle group

Sartorius

Gracilis

Vastus lateralis

Vastus medialis

Anterior tibial muscle group

Gastrocnemius

Front view of the human muscular system.

Extensors
of the wrist
and fingers

Triceps

Anterior
Middle Deltoid
Posterior

Trapezius

Infraspinatus

Latissimus
dorsi

Gluteus
maximus

Iliotibial
band

Trapezius

Hamstrings

Gastrocnemius

Achilles'
tendon

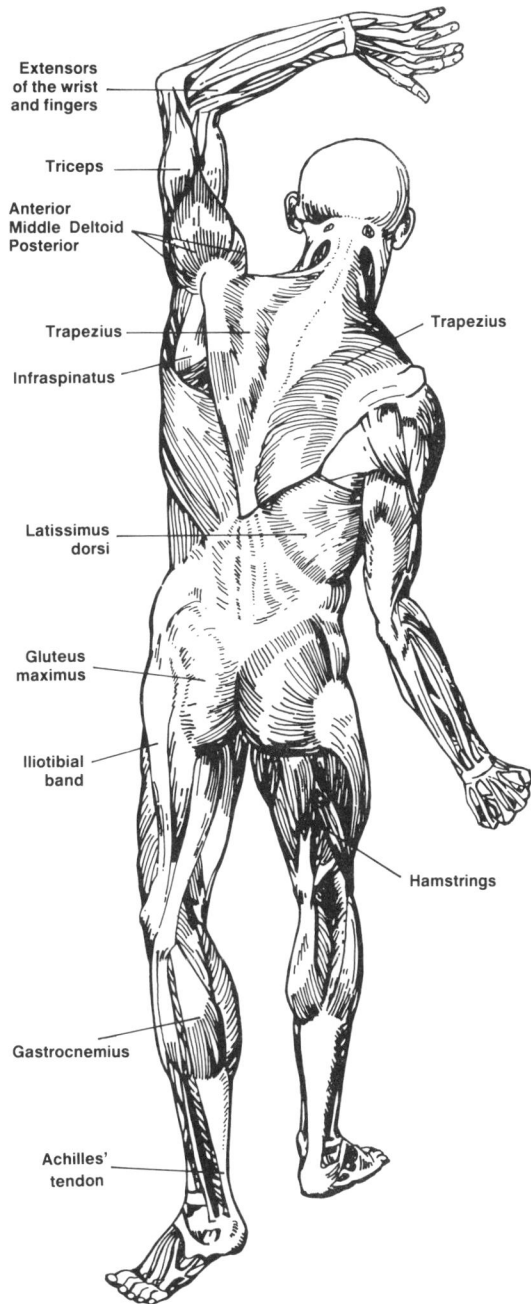

Back view of the human muscular system.

Tensor Fasciae Latae — arises from the front of the ilium near the hip and is inserted between two layers of fascia which continue down the outside of the thigh forming the iliotibial band, which in turn inserts itself into the outside of the upper tibia (shinbone).

Sartorius — the longest muscle in the body. Flat and narrow, it also arises from the front of the ilium, passes across the front of the thigh and inserts itself into the upper part of the inner surface of the tibia.

Adductors — a group of muscles on the inside of the thigh. They arise from the pubic bone and insert themselves at various points along the inside of the femur.

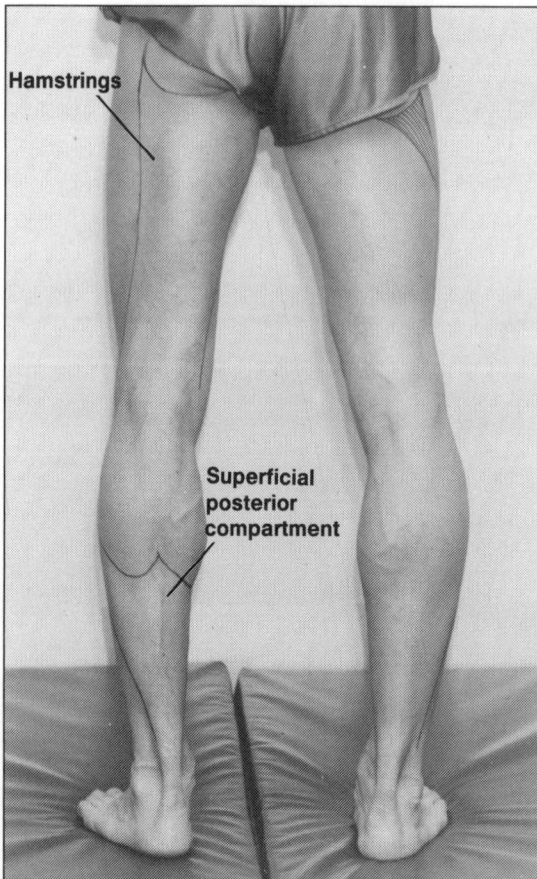

Fig. d

Hamstrings — a group of muscles at the back of the upper leg, including the *biceps femoris, semitendinosus,* and *semimembranosus.* (Fig. d)

Biceps femoris — as the name implies, *biceps femoris* has two parts. The 'long head' arises from the ischial tuberosity, while the 'short head' arises from an area at the back of the femur. The fibres of both heads converge to form a tendon which then divides into two parts and attaches to the upper tibia and fibula.

Semitendinosus — lies towards the centre of the hamstring group. It also arises from the ischial tuberosity, but attaches to the medial side of the tibia by way of a long tendon.

Semimembranosus — situated at the back and innerside of the thigh. It too arises from the ischial tuberosity and inserts itself by way of a long tendon onto the tibia.

Muscles of the gluteal region

The gluteal region (or the buttocks) contains nine individual muscles arranged in three layers. *Gluteus maximus* is the largest and, together with a portion of *gluteus medius*, forms the most superficial layer. All the muscles of the gluteal region arise from various parts of the coccyx, sacrum and ilium and insert themselves at various points around the greater trochanter of the femur. Most of the gluteus maximus also inserts into the iliotibial band.

Muscles of the lower back

There are two main muscle groups in the lower back — the lower part of the *erector spinae* group, which are the long, superficial muscles running lengthways up the back, parallel to the vertebrae, and the *quadratus lumborum*, beneath the erector spinae in the space between the bottom rib and the crest of the ilium, which also has attachments on the transverse processes of the last thoracic vertebrae and all five lumbar vertebrae.

Muscles of the lower leg

There are thirteen muscles within the lower leg. Depending upon their location and function they make up five muscle 'compartments' — the *anterior tibial*, the *lateral* or *peroneal*, the *superficial posterior*, the *deep posterior* compartment and the *tibialis posterior*. (Figs. e & f)

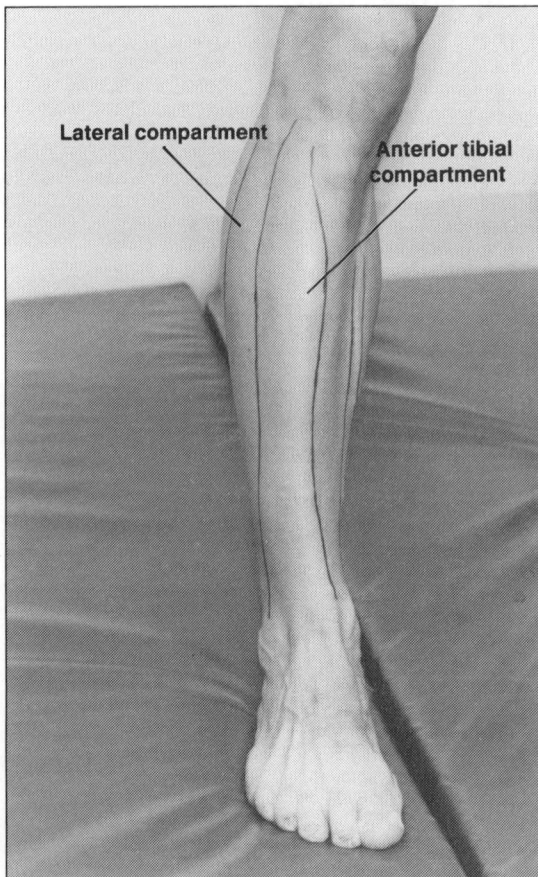

Fig. e

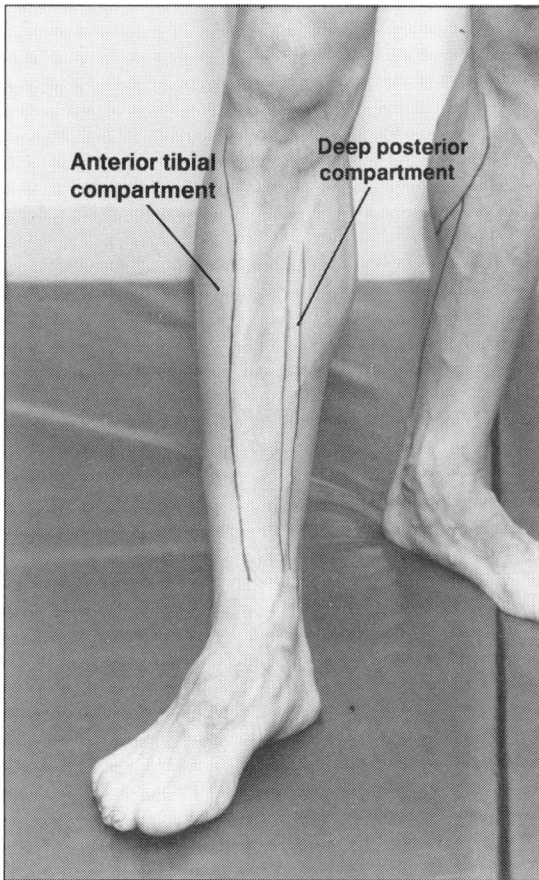

Fig. f

APPENDIX 2: STUDIES

Studies

Both people who practise massage and those who receive it regularly have no doubt that the manual manipulation of the body's soft tissues affords many benefits.

Eastern European countries have long recognised the value of massage and sports scientists in East Germany and the USSR in particular have undertaken extensive studies into its operation and effects. The information and knowledge gained from this research have resulted in massage practitioners playing an integral role in the development of many great East European athletes.

More recently an increasing number of similar studies have been made in Western countries, including some by the Australian Institute of Sport, looking at the effect massage has on athletic performance and the treatment of athletic injuries. We examine several such studies from both areas below.

1 'Changes in muscle and venous blood flow after massage'—Teriya, Praktika, Fizicheskoi, Kultery and Dubrovsky, 1982, Soviet Sports Review.

The authors state that heavy physical loads bring about an accumulation of metabolic products (wastes) and hypoxemia (a condition in which an inadequate amount of oxygen is available to or utilised by the body's tissues).

They found that the supply of oxygen and nutrients to tissues and the removal of waste products depends upon the intensity of muscle blood-flow and that at best only one-third of the capillaries in skeletal muscles are actually being used. (Where the capillaries branch off from metarterioles, there is a small ring of muscle known as the precapillary sphincter which can shut off the flow of blood to certain capillaries, allowing the blood to flow through the preferential channels.

When muscle blood supply is reduced, they note, the intensity of tissue metabolism decreases, 'which can have a great influence on the duration of the restorative processes'.

The authors studied the effect of massage on muscle and venous blood-flow, muscle tone and oxygen saturation of arterial blood in athletes. Twelve top-class athletes between twenty-two and twenty-seven years of age were used in these experiments.

Muscle blood-flow was measured using the 'Lassen method' and was examined in the tibialis anterior muscle of the lower leg.

A radioisotope, xenon, was injected into the muscle and intricate equipment was used to measure the clearance in millilitres per 100 grams in one minute of the xenon. The authors state that 'xenon clearance is directly proportional to muscle blood flow'.

The tests showed that muscle blood-flow before massage was 4.5 +/– 0.11 mililitres per 100 grams in one minute and 6.4 +/– 0.11 after massage, from which they concluded that massage *did* stimulate muscle blood-flow.

From further investigations the authors concluded that massage speeds up venous blood-flow and that the observed decrease in muscle tone (tightness) was caused by improved muscle blood-flow.

Their final conclusions were that 'massage can be used to relieve fatigue and increase physical work capacity in athletes'.

2 'Effects of massage in athletes with rotator cuff tendonitis'—Clews W. and Wajswelner H., 1988, Excel (A.I.S.) Vol. 4 No. 4.

'The shoulder joint is the focus of a wide range of sporting endeavour,' these researchers say. 'A strong, pain-free and flexible shoulder is essential to optimal performance in many sports including swimming, waterpolo, gymnastics, weightlifting and throwing.'

Athletes involved in these sports commonly suffer shoulder pain. Most are diagnosed as suffering from rotator cuff tendonitis, usually involving the 'long head' of biceps and supraspinatus tendons.

Pectoralis major and pectoralis minor, though not strictly part of the rotator cuff, were included in the study as athletes often report injury to these areas.

Clews and Wajswelner therefore decided to do 'a prospective study comparing the effectiveness of massage with that of ultrasound and placebo treatment, on reduction of pain and return of strength in the athletes suffering from rotator cuff tendonitis'.

Three groups of six subjects were chosen. All were elite athletes involved in either swimming, waterpolo, gymnastics or a throwing sport and were diagnosed as having rotator cuff tendonitis, displaying unilateral signs (pain in only one shoulder).

The three groups were designated A, B and C. All performed a standard pre-test on the first day of the experiment, involving measurement of maximal isometric force production (which the researchers called the strength test) on both arms and measurement of pain produced during the strength test on the injured arm only.

A visual analogue pain scale was used to measure the pain produced during the strength test. Here the subjects were asked to rate their pain from zero (no pain at all) to ten (the worst pain imaginable).

Following these tests all subjects began three consecutive days of treatment. Group A received fifteen minutes' standard form of massage, ice treatment and anti-inflammatory medication. Group B received fifteen minutes of pulsed ultrasound therapy, ice treatment and anti-inflammatory medication. Group C received fifteen minutes of 'sham' ultrasound (the machine was not switched on), ice treatment and anti-inflammatory medication.

All subjects had their strength and levels of pain retested on day three of the experiment, following the last treatment session.

In this study the authors found that pain was considerably reduced in all three groups. However, there was no significant difference in the effect of massage, ultrasound and 'placebo' treatments on relieving pain. It is possible that pain was affected mainly by the non-mechanical therapies such as the ice and anti-inflammatory medication.

It was considered necessary to have all subjects use ice and anti-inflammatory medication in order to achieve the earliest possible return to their normal training regimen.

However, the results and analysis did show that both ultrasound and massage had a beneficial effect in terms of strength gains, which was significantly different to gains made with 'placebo' treatment.

On average, the subjects who received massage or ultrasound treatment improved 11.6 per cent more than those who received 'placebo' treatment, when tested for maximal isometric force production following three days of treatment.

All subjects continued full training during the course of the experiment. The authors conclude that massage is a valuable adjunct to the treatment of rotator cuff tendonitis in high level athletes.

3 'The effects of massage to the hamstring muscle group on range of motion'—Crosman, Chateavert and Weisberg, 1984, Journal of Orthopaedic and Sports Physical Therapy.

The authors state that 'limitation in the range of motion of the hamstring muscle group has the potential for increasing the risk of athletic injury ... It can be said that hamstring tightness can be either a predisposing factor in traumatic injuries, or can result from a variety of pathological conditions from which further compensations may result'.

(Further to this, Kuprian states in *Physical Therapy for Sports 1981* that 'any passive or active activity that promotes stretching of muscles will aid in the prevention of sports related injuries').

Thirty-four female volunteers between the ages of eighteen and thirty-five took part in the experiment.

A standard goniometer was used to measure passive knee extension and hip flexion in a straight-leg raise. An additional measurement was made from the lateral malleolus (the bony prominence on the outside of the ankle) to the massage table at the end of the passive range of a straight-leg raise.

Each subject had one of her legs assigned to the test group and the other to the control group, so that while hamstring flexibility was measured on both legs, only one leg received massage treatment.

Measurements of flexibility were taken immediately before and immediately after massage treatment, and again seven days later.

A standardised massage treatment lasting nine to twelve minutes was performed on the test group. It was a 'double-blind' experiment, meaning that the researcher who performed the flexibility measurements did not perform the massage treatments, nor was he aware of which legs had received massage. This step was taken simply to rule out any possible bias in the procedure governing the flexibility measurements.

All subjects continued with their normal exercise and stretching routines during the one-week test period. Pretreatment, post treatment and seven days' post treatment scores of range of motion or flexibility were obtained for both treatment and control legs of each subject. The scores were compared for each subject and the differences used for statistical analysis.

The results showed a 'definite association between the massaged test legs and an increase in range of motion'. The researchers also found that the range of motion of most subjects tended to return to the pretreatment state during a seven-day period following the massage.

The authors therefore conclude that 'massage is an effective means for increasing range of motion and should be an integral part of patient care'.

4 'The influence of repeated massage on leg strength'—Carter, Zhang, Minikin, and Telford, 1988, Proceedings of National Scientific Conference, Australian Sports Medicine Federation.

Weightlifters in top-class competition need enormous leg strength and power. The purpose of this study was to determine whether massage influences the recovery and/or adaptation of the knee extensor and flexor muscle groups during two weeks of intensive training.

The subjects were eight junior weightlifters between sixteen and seventeen years of age, training at the Australian Institute of Sport. The subjects were randomly divided into a treatment and a control group.

For two weeks the treatment group received traditional Chinese massage administered for one hour daily, which incorporated point pressure, kneading and friction. The control group received 'sham' ultrasound therapy, which served as a 'placebo' treatment. For the second period of two weeks the treatment groups were reversed.

Throughout the course of the study both groups of weightlifters were tested for knee extensor and flexor strength using a Cybex isokinetic dynamometer. Statistical analysis of the data showed that while receiving massage treatment they made significant gains in leg strength, with no significant change being evident when receiving 'placebo' treatment.

The authors concluded that, through facilitating quicker recovery, daily massage treatment helped the weightlifters adapt to two weeks of intensive training.

5 'Effects of therapeutic massage vs. physiotherapy modalities on interstitial compartment pressure'—Hannaford, Clews, Fardy and Wajswelner, 1988, Proceedings of National Scientific Conference, Australian Sports Medicine Federation.

The information collected from this continuing study strongly supports the use of massage in the treatment of compartment pressure syndrome and gives rise to some interesting theories on the efficacy of massage.

As we have seen in the section on the muscular system, there are a number of connective tissue structures associated with the muscles. Many muscle groups, particularly those of the lower limbs, are enveloped in a connective tissue called fascia.

Within the lower leg there are thirteen individual muscles which are classified in groups according to where they are situated about the tibia and fibula and the functions or actions they perform. Each group has its own covering of fascia and is referred to as a muscle compartment.

The lower leg is generally considered to consist of four muscle compartments. However, Davey and his colleagues ('The Tibialis Posterior Muscle Compartment') found evidence indicating the presence of a fifth compartment.

A patient with lower leg compartment pressure syndrome will complain of tightness and pain occurring with exercise. There will often be weakness and tenderness in the muscles and oedema (swelling) will also frequently be present.

A major factor in compartment pressure syndrome is that while the muscle will become enlarged during exercise, mainly due to increased blood flow, the enveloping fascia does not have similar properties by which to expand and accommodate the muscles. This results in an increase in compartment pressure.

A surgical procedure called fasciotomy is commonly prescribed for patients suffering from compartment pressure syndrome. It involves an open incision of the fascia along the length of the muscle compartment.

A co-author observed that patients showing symptoms consistent with those of compartment pressure syndrome responded favourably to massage treatment. It was therefore decided to undertake a research project. The subjects were volunteers exhibiting bilateral compartment pressure syndrome of the anterior tibialis compartment, which was confirmed by a pressure test taken after exercise.

Compartment pressures can be measured using an indwelling slit catheter. The equipment used in this study consists of a relatively large hollow needle which is inserted into the muscle compartment under local anaesthetic. A plastic tube connected to a pressure gauge is fed through the needle into the muscle compartment. The needle is removed, leaving one end of the tube within the compartment. A resisted isometric contraction is performed to confirm that the target area has been reached. This results in an immediate elevation of intra-compartmental pressure as shown on the pressure gauge. Pressure readings are taken in millimetres of mercury (mm/hg). The normal range of pressure is 0–10mm/hg.

The subjects were randomly assigned to one of two treatment groups. Group one received massage treatment — ten minutes on each leg per treatment. Group two received physiotherapy modality treatment — ultrasound, magnetic field and interferential.

The treatment schedule for the two groups was identical, involving treatment on five consecutive days for the first week and alternate days for the following three weeks. Compartment pressure testing was performed before and after the initial treatment session, at the completion of the fourth week and finally at the end of the tenth week, following a six-week period during which the subjects received no treatment at all.

In both treatment groups there was a reduction over time in interstitial compartment pressure. Subjects treated with physiotherapy modalities showed the greatest pressure differential between the first day of treatment and the fifth, whereas in the massage group the greatest differential occurred during the period of the initial treatment. Both groups exhibited a trend towards the normal pressure of 10mm/hg, with the massage group attaining readings around this level sooner than the physiotherapy group.

At the end of ten weeks all the subjects were engaged in their normal sport at their usual level and frequency. None of them was considered to have sufficient symptoms to warrant surgery.

At this stage the authors conclude that both physiotherapy modalities and massage are associated with a subjective improvement in the pain of exertional compartment pressure syndromes and a drop in interstitial compartment pressure towards normal.

While improvements resulting from massage treatment have been objectively measured, the physiological changes which have resulted from the massage treatment are still unclear. The study has given rise to a number of theories relating to the efficacy of massage in the treatment of compartment pressure syndrome. These include:

- Massage returns muscles to their optimal resting length with a subsequent reduction in the circumference of muscle mass.

- Massage assists the functioning of the lymphatic system in the removal of local oedema.

- The mechanical action of massage will free adhesions between fascia and muscle mass, leaving the fascia more pliable.

- Massage increases muscle blood-flow and with this comes an increase in the interchange of nourishment and waste products between the circulatory system and muscle tissue.

The most relevant point is that a condition for which surgery is commonly prescribed appears to respond at least symptomatically, to both physiotherapy modalities and massage treatment.

At the end of their involvement in the study, all subjects were instructed in self-massage techniques as represented in this book and to date have been able to maintain their improved condition through their own endeavours.

In summary, these examples of scientific research add weight to our belief that massage should play an integral role in the development of your athletic prowess.

Through the prevention and treatment of soft-tissue injuries and the promotion of recovery and adaptation during intense training periods, massage can assist you in reaching your real potential and achieving your goals and ambitions, whether they be in the international competitive arena or merely your local park as part of your personal program to achieve health and fitness.

Further reading

The Magic of Massage
Ouida West
Delilah Communications, USA

Runner's World Massage Book
Ray Hosler
Runner's World Books, USA

Athletic Massage
Rich Phaigh and Paul Perry
Simon & Schuster, USA

The Muscle Fitness Book
Francine St George,
Simon & Schuster, Australia

INDEX

Index